Psychotherap
and Medicatio

Psychoanalytic Inquiry Book Series

Volume 22

Psychotherapy *and* Medication

The Challenge of Integration

Fredric N. Busch and Larry S. Sandberg

The Analytic Press
Taylor & Francis Group
New York London

The Analytic Press
Taylor & Francis Group
270 Madison Avenue
New York, NY 10016

The Analytic Press
Taylor & Francis Group
27 Church Road
Hove, East Sussex BN3 2FA

Printed in the United States of America on acid-free paper
10 9 8 7 6 5 4 3 2 1

International Standard Book Number-13: 978-0-88163-451-8 (Hardcover)

Library of Congress Cataloging-in-Publication Data

Busch, Fredric, 1958-
Psychotherapy and medication : the challenge of integration / Fredric N. Busch and Larry S. Sandberg.
p. ; cm. -- (Psychoanalytic inquiry book series ; 22)
Includes bibliographical references and index.
ISBN-13: 978-0-88163-451-8 (hardcover : alk. paper)
ISBN-10: 0-88163-451-4 (hardcover : alk. paper)
1. Mental illness--Chemotherapy. 2. Combined modality therapy. 3. Psychotherapy. I. Sandberg, Larry S. II. Title. III. Series.
[DNLM: 1. Psychotherapy. 2. Combined Modality Therapy--adverse effects. 3. Drug Therapy--adverse effects. 4. Transference (Psychology) W1 PS427F v.22 2007 / WM 420 B977p 2007]

RC483.B87 2007
616.89'14061--dc22 2007001395

Visit the Taylor & Francis Web site at
http://www.taylorandfrancis.com

and The Analytic Press Web site at
http://www.analyticpress.com

We dedicate this book to our fathers:

Dr. Harris Busch, who inspired a search for better ways to help others, and

Murray Sandberg, who, with love and sacrifice, encouraged his children to realize their dreams.

Contents

The Authors

Fredric N. Busch is a clinical associate professor of psychiatry at Weill Cornell Medical College and a faculty member of the Columbia University Center for Psychoanalytic Training and Research. He is also on the editorial board of *Psychoanalytic Inquiry*. Dr. Busch has authored over 30 publications as well as 10 books or book chapters. His writing and research have focused on the links between psychoanalysis and psychiatry, including psychodynamic approaches to specific disorders, psychoanalytic research, and psychoanalysis and medication. He has coauthored three books on the psychoanalytic approach to specific disorders: *Manual of Panic Focused Psychodynamic Psychotherapy*, *Psychodynamic Approaches to the Adolescent With Panic Disorder*, and *Psychodynamic Treatment of Depression*.

Dr. Busch has been involved in research on panic-focused psychodynamic psychotherapy, including the first study to demonstrate efficacy of psychodynamic treatment of panic disorder, recently published in the *American Journal of Psychiatry*. Additionally, he has written on integrating the theoretical conceptualizations and clinical approaches of psychoanalytic treatments and medication. This has included coediting an issue of *Psychoanalytic Inquiry* on this topic and coauthoring two seminal papers on "treatment triangles" addressing the complex interactions of the psychotherapist, psychopharmacologist, and patient.

Larry S. Sandberg is a clinical associate professor of psychiatry at Weill Cornell Medical Center and lecturer in psychiatry at Columbia University Center for Psychoanalytic Training and Research. He has a long-standing interest in interdisciplinary studies and psychoanalysis and a particular interest in psychotherapy, psychoanalysis, and medication. Dr. Sandberg has been instrumental in creating a course on the integration of psychotherapy, psychoanalysis, and medication for psychoanalytic candidates at Columbia and has been invited to teach it to psychiatric residents at the New York University School of Medicine. He has presented on this topic at national and local psychoanalytic meetings as well as contributed to the literature in the form of papers, book reviews, and letters. He is also involved in research on panic-focused psychodynamic psychotherapy. Dr. Sandberg maintains a private practice in psychoanalysis and adult psychiatry.

Acknowledgment

We would like to acknowledge Dr. Paul Stepansky for his editorial assistance.

1

Introduction

Over the last 20 years the use of medication in combination with psychodynamic psychotherapy or psychoanalysis has shifted from an infrequent occurrence to common practice (Roose, 1995). Paralleling this shift, attitudes toward medication have changed from viewing this intervention as disruptive or an addition of last resort to a welcome aid to the analytic process. This rapid change, however, has created difficulty, both theoretically and technically, in the integration of medication use into the analytic setting (Busch, 1998; Roose & Johannet, 1998). Although these treatments can work well together, there are potential pitfalls that can disrupt the effectiveness of combining treatments. The intent of this book is to provide information on how to work with medication theoretically, clinically, and technically in the context of a psychodynamic or psychoanalytic treatment. Toward this goal, we will describe the evidence that this change has taken place, examine the factors that have led to this shift, and review the issues and questions about combining these treatments.

PSYCHOANALYSTS' SHIFTING VIEWS OF MEDICATIONS

Early concerns about the use of medication in a psychoanalytic treatment focused on several issues (Roose, 1995). Psychoanalysts feared that medication would reduce motivation for change by easing negative feelings that led patients to pursue treatment. In addition, anxiety was believed to be of particular value because it indicated the presence of psychic conflict, thus aiding the analyst in pursuing the unconscious sources of the patient's symptoms. In this sense, the presence or onset of anxiety could be looked at as a positive sign rather than a detriment because it suggested that conflicts were being addressed. Since anxiety was an indicator of conflict rather than a cause of the patient's problems, it was not necessary to treat it with medication. In addition to potentially derailing valuable negative affects, medications were seen as possibly undermining the patient's sense of autonomy and self-esteem (Sarwer-Foner, 1983).

Because medications were viewed as containing significant risks for treatment, they were typically relegated to a secondary role, even by pioneers in introducing medication to psychoanalysis. Ostow (1962) saw medication only as a support for psychoanalysis, warning that "drugs should not be used in psychoanalysis or psychotherapy unless they are essential to protect the patient or to protect the treatment" (p. 147). As late as 1983 Sarwer-Foner stated,

> It is clear that one will not give pharmacotherapy to a patient unless one believes that the symptoms the patient presents and the disease process producing the symptoms *cannot be mastered or dealt with by the patient in psychotherapy at that moment in time or space*. If this assumption is not correct—if the patient can, in fact, with the help of the physician, correct and master the intrapsychic problems causing the symptoms and the suffering—then the psychotropic medication ... is not really needed ... (p. 167). The patient may perceive the act of taking the medicine as proof that he cannot handle his symptoms or problems without it. (p. 168)

By the mid 1980s, however, psychoanalysts began to talk increasingly about potential benefits of medications (Cooper, 1985; Esman, 1989; Lipton, 1983). Recent studies (Donovan & Roose, 1995; Roose & Stern, 1995; Yang et al., 2004) highlight a shift in both frequency of and attitude toward medication use. In a study at Columbia University Center for Psychoanalytic Training and Research with a return rate of 89% (Roose & Stern, 1995), candidates were given an anonymous questionnaire to evaluate their level of medication use. The study found that 29% of the candidates' cases in analysis were also on medication (16/56) and that 11 of 24 of the candidates (46%) had at least one patient in analysis who was also on medication.

To test the theory that this was just a trend in the younger generation of analysts, the researchers then assessed training and supervising analysts (Donovan & Roose, 1995). Of those surveyed, 76% returned the questionnaire regarding patients they had had in analysis in the preceding 5 years. The analysts reported on 277 patients: 18% (51/277) had been on medication during psychoanalysis, and 62% (21/34) of analysts had at least one patient who received medication. In 84% of cases (36/43) in which patients had been given medication for a mood disorder, the psychoanalysts noted that the mood disorder as well as the psychoanalytic process improved. Indicating that Columbia is not the only institute demonstrating this trend, graduate analysts at the Cincinnati Psychoanalytic Institute were found to have 36% of their patients in analysis on medication (Cabaniss & Roose, 2005).

FACTORS LEADING TO INCREASED MEDICATION USE

Several factors have combined to bring about this attitudinal shift in psychoanalysts regarding medication use. The availability of safer, better tolerated medications has reduced the adverse impact that medications may have in treatment. In addition, systematic studies have repeatedly confirmed the effectiveness of medication for a variety of syndromes, providing a strong evidentiary basis regarding their use (Janicek et al., 2006). Third, multiple external pressures have affected psychiatrists and psychoanalysts in ways that call for more medication use, such as insurance company oversight, pharmaceutical company marketing, and direct-to-consumer advertising. Finally, the boundaries between the biological and psychological bases of syndromes have become increasingly unclear. For example, syndromes previously viewed as psychologically based or as personality disorders have been redefined as primarily biological illnesses found to be responsive to medication. Important examples include dysthymic disorder (Kocsis et al., 1988, 1996), formerly characterized as depressive personality, and attention deficit disorder (Wender, 1995), in which the individual exhibits difficulties with procrastination, concentration, and attention previously seen as passive–aggressive or as derived from psychic conflict.

Another factor that has played a role has been the shift to evidence-based medicine, which expounds the view that treatments should be prescribed according to whether they have demonstrated efficacy in treatment of specific disorders. The gold standard for these determinations is randomized, controlled clinical trials in which the treatment, delivered in a form in which adherence can be assessed, is compared to a placebo. Medication and certain psychotherapies have been extensively studied using these approaches, but psychoanalytic treatments have not.

In the late 1980s the stakes were raised in the lawsuit of *Osheroff v. Chestnut Lodge*, in which a patient sued Chestnut Lodge Hospital for treating his depressive disorder with an intense inpatient psychoanalytically oriented psychotherapy instead of medication. Klerman, a consultant to the plaintiff in this case, stated that "this case goes a long way to establishing the patient's right to effective treatment" (1990, p. 416), by which he meant treatment found to be effective through controlled clinical trials. In addition, Klerman warned that "the courts may be an appropriate arena for litigation when a small minority of the profession persist in practices that scientific evidence and professional judgment have deemed obsolete" (p. 417).

Stone (1990) wrote a strong rebuttal to Klerman's comments, noting that Klerman (1988) had stated in his writing that "individual psychotherapy based on psychodynamic principles remains the most widely used form of psychotherapy. Although systematic, controlled, clinical studies do not exist, clinical experience supports the value of this form of treatment" (p. 330). In spite of this response, some psychoanalysts interpreted the *Osheroff* debate as creating legal pressure to consider and employ medication.

As Stone averred, "Klerman's recommendations may have considerable legal consequences, even if his ideas have no basis in law and are intended only as clinical recommendations" (p. 420).

Studies showing an advantage in combined treatment of many disorders compared to medication or psychotherapy given alone (Barlow, Gorman, Shear, & Woods, 2000; Keller et al., 2000; Thase, 2000) have also influenced prescribing trends among psychoanalysts—despite the primary use of interpersonal psychotherapy or cognitive–behavioral therapy rather than psychoanalytic treatment in these studies. In depressive disorders, combination treatment has been found to be particularly valuable for more severe episodes, whereas milder symptoms often respond to psychotherapy or pharmacotherapy alone (Thase et al., 1997). A more recent study of chronic depression demonstrated a significant additional benefit for combined treatment over medication (nefazodone) or psychotherapy (a form of cognitive behavior therapy) alone (Keller et al., 2000).

Recommendations for providing psychotherapy plus medication in at least some cases have been made for a variety of disorders (American Psychiatric Association, 1998, 2000). For example, the practice guideline for the treatment of patients with panic disorder refers to a study in which the addition of psychodynamic psychotherapy to a medication treatment reduced the risk of relapse. The guideline avers that "psychodynamic psychotherapy is commonly used in conjunction with medication on the basis of a clinical consensus that it is effective for some patients" (American Psychiatric Association, 1998, p. 21). Based on studies and clinical experience, recommendations for combined treatment are frequently made for patients with more severe depression or anxiety disorders, patients who are unresponsive to psychotherapy or pharmacotherapy alone, or patients who have problems complying with treatment. The revised practice guideline for the treatment of patients with major depressive disorder states:

> The combination of a specific effective psychotherapy and medication may be a useful initial treatment choice for patients with psychosocial issues, interpersonal problems, or a comorbid axis II disorder together with moderate to severe major depressive disorder. In addition, patients who have had a history of only partial response to adequate trials of single-treatment modalities may benefit from combined treatment. Poor adherence with treatments may also warrant combined treatment with pharmacotherapy and psychotherapeutic approaches that focus on treatment adherence. (American Psychiatric Association, 2000, p. 9)

POSITIVES AND PITFALLS FOR PSYCHOANALYSTS IN THE USE OF MEDICATION

There are many benefits for psychoanalysts and their patients in bringing medication into their therapeutic armamentarium (addressed in greater depth in chapter 5). Chief among these is the potential to relieve patients more rapidly of distressing and impairing symptoms. Medication treatment can often aid patients in engaging in psychotherapy—for example, by reducing disruptions in concentration and motivation. Rather than erasing anxiety that can be useful for psychoanalytic exploration, medication can help to reduce the anxiety to tolerable levels that can allow more effective engagement of the patient's observing ego. Exploration of the meanings of medication and being medicated can provide an additional window into a patient's intrapsychic life, conflicts, and transference reactions and help patients comply with their medication. When a therapist is working with another practitioner who is prescribing medication, a positive collaborative relationship can provide additional support and perspective for treatment.

However, potential pitfalls in medicating patients also exist. Psychoanalysts can experience a disruption in their analytic stance as they attempt to assess the patient systematically with regard to indications for and reactions and response to medications. Preexisting negative attitudes toward medication, conscious or unconscious, may affect the analysts' abilities to think about medication psychodynamically. A recent review of the charts of candidates in analytic training indicated little or no documentation of medication assessment or monitoring, as well as minimal or no comment about the impact of the medication on the status of the transference and countertransference (Cabaniss & Roose, 2005). When an analyst is working with another practitioner who is prescribing medication, conflicts can develop that can disrupt or adversely affect the treatment (see chapter 7).

In addition to problems for the analyst, medication can create difficulties for patients in analysis or psychodynamic psychotherapy. They may experience discussions about medication as intrusive or have concerns that the analyst sees them as too "sick" for analysis alone. Symptom relief through medication can reduce some patients' interest in addressing broader intrapsychic and interpersonal problems and lead them to discontinue the analytic treatment.

PSYCHODYNAMIC PSYCHOTHERAPY VERSUS PSYCHOANALYSIS AND THE USE OF MEDICATION

Conducting inquiry and treatment of patients with medication is more complex for patients in psychoanalysis than for those in psychodynamic psychotherapy. Psychoanalysis will typically include fewer directive interventions, less give and take between analyst and patient, and a lower frequency of nonanalytic interventions than psychodynamic psychotherapy, and therefore the interventions required for psychopharmacological evaluation and monitoring will be more discontinuous and potentially disruptive.

In conducting psychoanalysis then, a psychoanalyst will more strongly consider employing a split treatment to minimize disruption to the analysis and will be very alert to the impact of medicating on the analytic process and the transference. In this book, there will not be a specific chapter on combining treatments in psychoanalysis versus psychodynamic psychotherapy, but in certain instances we will point out special factors involved in employing medication during psychoanalysis.

QUESTIONS ABOUT COMBINED TREATMENT ADDRESSED IN THIS BOOK

As this overview suggests, in spite of the increasing willingness of psychoanalysts to combine medication and psychoanalysis or psychodynamic psychotherapy, many questions about providing this treatment lack definitive answers.

How can we best integrate these treatments, theoretically and clinically (chapter 2)?
How do we initially introduce medication to patients (chapter 3)?
What can be gained from exploring the meanings of and transference issues with prescribing medications (chapter 4)?
What are the clinical advantages of combined treatment (chapter 5)?
What is the impact of medication discussions and prescribing on the analyst's role and how is this best handled (chapter 6)?
In situations in which the analyst is a psychiatrist, should the analyst prescribe the medication or hand the task to another physician (chapter 6)?
If two practitioners are involved in treatment, how do they best handle their relationship with each other and the patient (chapter 7)?
How does understanding the dynamics of anxiety and depressive disorders aid with managing combined treatment (chapter 8)?
How do we address combined treatment in complex cases (chapter 9)?

This book will evolve a framework, based on current evidence and clinical experience, as to how to best answer these questions.

2

Theoretical Bases of Combined Treatment

As outlined in chapter 1, psychodynamic therapists and psychoanalysts have increasingly turned to pharmacotherapy as a valuable tool in their clinical armamentarium. It is important to therapist and patient alike to have an understanding of the rationale for combined treatment. The theoretical stance of the therapist will significantly affect his way of speaking to his patient and giving care; that is, his orientation vis-à-vis combined treatment will have an impact on *how* treatment is combined, not only *if* it is combined. Inherent in the notion of combined treatment is a view of the human mind as complex and of the therapeutic endeavor as similarly complex. The clinician's capacity to consider combined treatment is itself a powerful antidote to the dangers of reductionism. Also, combined treatment, by its very nature, invites numerous questions about the nature of suffering that can be complicated by falsely dichotomous thinking. Among the common if not universal questions raised are: Is the illness biological or psychological? Is the problem in the genes or was it caused by stress? Is it the person or his brain? Unless the clinician has considered these questions, he will not be able to explore them constructively with his patient.

In this chapter, we will first examine the theoretical basis within psychoanalysis and dynamic psychotherapy for combined treatment by turning to Freud and to other analysts who have contributed on the topic. We will discuss early attempts within psychoanalysis to understand combined treatment based on a two-illness model, assessing its advantages and disadvantages. The recent integrative efforts of Kendler (2005) will be elucidated as a way of providing the clinician with a comprehensive theoretical and philosophical framework for combined treatment that moves beyond the more rudimentary two-illness model. Such a framework is necessary to accommodate interactional models that capture the complex dialectic that takes place in trying to combine treatment empathically and competently. The application of more complex models to the clinical situation will be shown to require an inevitable oscillation between different ways of relating (Cabaniss, 1998; Sandberg, 1998).

PERSPECTIVES FROM WITHIN PSYCHOANALYSIS

In chapter 1, the basis for the antagonism of dynamic therapists and analysts toward the use of medication was elaborated. There was a rigid adherence to rules of technique that made the use of medication relatively or absolutely contraindicated. Psychic determinism was embraced reductionistically. In the context of these tendencies to exclude the relevance of biological factors, it is important to be reminded that Freudian theory has always accommodated the role of the body as an essential consideration of mental life. Freud's core concept of instinct as existing on the frontier between the mental and the somatic illustrates this. Furthermore, his view of the ego as first and foremost a body ego and his conceptualization of a complementary series reflected an awareness that development always included an interplay between constitutional and environmental factors. Freud's acceptance of the limitations of psychoanalysis and his anticipation of other therapeutics are well known (Freud, 1938):

> But here we are concerned with therapy only insofar as it works by psychological means; and for the time being we have no other. The future may teach us to exercise a direct influence, by means of particular substances, on the amounts of energy and their distribution in the mental apparatus. It may be that there are still undreamt-of possibilities of therapy. (p. 182)

While this quote is often seen in papers on pharmacotherapy and psychoanalysis to remind analysts that Freud anticipated advances in drug treatment, it is important to highlight the explicit biological/somatic point of view as essential and irreducible.

Although Heinz Hartmann's ego psychology is now considered part of a bygone era (Bergman, 2000), his writings also provide an explicit and heuristically useful conceptual basis for combined treatment from within psychoanalysis. Hartmann (1939) believed that the mind has areas of functioning that are autonomous and not primarily derived from conflict (affect regulation, impulse control, and attention, for example), yet could become secondarily entangled in conflict. For many psychoanalysts the concept of ego functions operating independently of conflict was the antithesis of a truly psychoanalytic view that emphasized the inevitably conflicted state of the mind. Yet, an important implication of the notion of autonomous ego functions is that they permit a way of thinking about the role of pharmacotherapy in psychoanalysis: Some patients may be viewed as having impairments in autonomous ego function that could be ameliorated through the use of medication.

Besides Freud and Hartmann, other analysts have looked at how biological factors interact with psychoanalytic models of the mind, but this approach has not been emphasized in the psychoanalytic literature (Cornell, 1985). Kandel (1999) laments the decline of psychoanalysis as not having evolved scientifically in recent decades, in part because it has failed to recognize itself as a branch of biology. While offering the opinion that psychoanalysis embodies the most coherent view of mind, he opined that a dialogue was essential between psychoanalysis and biology in order to achieve a coherent understanding of mind. Combined treatment necessitates and facilitates such a dialogue.

The Two-Illness Model

Whereas the earliest efforts to combine treatment relied heavily on translating drug action into metapsychological terms (Ostow, 1962), subsequent efforts shifted away from this approach and attempted to find the points of intersection that Kandel has encouraged. Psychoanalysts began entertaining multiple models of the mind (Kantor, 1990) or suggesting more pragmatic treatment approaches based on evidence (Roose, 1990), thereby attempting to create a theoretical space in which to consider the usefulness of pharmacotherapy.

Kantor (1990) encouraged a two-illness model. He put forth the idea that some patients would be helped by considering that they suffered from character problems that would benefit from psychoanalysis and depressive illness that could be ameliorated by medication. He described a view of comorbidity in which one illness was psychological and in need of psychoanalysis or psychotherapy and one illness was deemed biological and in need of somatic treatment.

Although the two-illness model was itself an oversimplification, Kantor was attempting to deal with a reductionistic attitude on the part of many analysts who resisted embracing an integrative pluralism that would make it acceptable to turn to medication while engaging in analysis. Furthermore, he was highlighting a well-known clinical fact: Patients who are deeply depressed are unable to make use of what psychoanalysis has to offer, due to disruptions in ego functions. Pollock (1986) posited a similar two-illness model, when he asked, "Do multiple psychological diseases exist simultaneously?" He focused on the growing scientific literature supporting the genetic risk factors for bipolar disease and viewed this as evidence that a biological condition can exist alongside essentially neurotic symptomatology. Again, patients could be suffering from two illnesses simultaneously (biological and psychological), thus warranting two different approaches (medication and psychoanalysis).

Advantages of a Two-Illness Model

Contemporary models shy away from this kind of reductionism, but a two-illness model has certain values. Brain-to-mind causality and the legitimacy of alternative, nondynamic models of the mind become a part of the analyst's theorizing. Given the substantial comorbidity that exists in actual clinical practice for psychoanalysts and psychodynamic clinicians (Doidge et al., 2002; Friedman et al., 2005), this two-illness model remains helpful in guiding the clinician to consider the possibility that another illness that is not primarily psychological exists, which may benefit from medication.

Mr. A presented for treatment having relocated from another part of the country, where he was diagnosed and treated for recurrent manic episodes characterized by grandiosity, impulsive spending, and impaired judgment. He had become noncompliant with his lithium treatment after his first episode and soon thereafter suffered a relapse requiring hospitalization. By the time he came to treatment he expressed a clear awareness of the risk of recurrent illness, having "learned his lesson," and firmly believed that whatever was lost with regard to the pleasure of an elated mood was more than offset by not damaging the professional and personal areas of his life through his manic behavior. He acknowledged the genetic loading within his own family and felt that a biological explanation made sense. Over the subsequent decade, Mr. A would visit every 4 to 6 months as a way of monitoring his mood, checking his lithium level and thyroid functions. He consistently expressed the belief that lithium was a "lifesaver" for him.

However, he twice entered psychotherapy for a period of a year or so. In one instance, it was to discuss his frustrating relationship with his girlfriend, who was also his business partner. On a second occasion, it was to express his worries about his son, who as an adolescent had developed a substance-abuse problem and exhibited manic-type symptoms. In both periods of brief psychotherapy, narcissistic and dependent issues were a focus. In the first period, the psychiatrist explored how, on the one hand, Mr. A felt entitled to have more of a commitment from his girlfriend, while, on the other hand, his fears of dependency created a preference for a more aloof relationship. In the second instance, he needed help to make less use of denial so that he could mobilize on his son's behalf. The fact that he suffered from recurrent mania was relevant only insofar as the illness affected his self-esteem and dependency fears. The bipolar disorder itself was considered to be a biological illness effectively treated by his use of lithium carbonate.

Disadvantages of a Two-Illness Model

While the two-illness model is helpful in certain clinical situations, concealed within the model is a risky reductionism of its own. Insofar as certain conditions are conceptualized as brain-based disorders that require somatic treatment, there is little room to consider psychotherapy or psychoanalysis unless a second illness (typically character pathology) is posited. Current research in combined treatment (Thase, 2003) indicates that the most robust findings for the efficacy of combined treatment are for the disorders most typically thought of as brain based (major depression, for example); that is, medication and psychotherapy combine to treat the one illness. While this research typically involves nonpsychodynamic psychotherapies, psychoanalysts often find psychodynamic exploration useful in treating such disorders.

Ms. B presented for treatment having seen a drug advertisement for the use of Zoloft (sertraline) to treat panic disorder that described its mechanism of action as "correcting a chemical imbalance." She described a long history of panic attacks with accompanying symptoms of agoraphobia. She had an enmeshed relationship with her mother that complicated her relationships with men, none of whom met her mother's standards. An intensification of her panic attacks was correlated with problems in her current relationship. The patient was disturbed by her anxiety symptoms, which left her with an imminent fear of death. Efforts to engage her introspectively were met with incredulity and defensiveness, with her asserting the legitimacy of her "chemical imbalance." The clinician, while suggesting a complex etiology for her symptoms, prescribed the desired drug, which markedly diminished her panic symptoms with much gratitude expressed by the patient; she continued to report little distress about her enmeshed relationship with her mother and even less motivation to explore her difficulties in sustaining a healthy relationship with a man.

This case illustrates how patients are at risk of seizing upon their need for medication as evidence of a brain disease without psychological cause or meaning. Some patients, however, are satisfied with relief of symptoms provided by medication and may not desire additional psychotherapeutic treatment for psychological problems.

We suggest that the discovery of comorbidity marks a starting point rather than an endpoint in the clinical decision-making process. In a recent effectiveness study of psychiatrist/analysts, Friedman, Garrison, Bucci, and Gorman (2005) found that 59% of patients treated in long-term psychotherapy/analysis had both Axis I and Axis II disorders, whereas only 11% had Axis II disorders alone. When comorbidity exists, the clinician needs to consider his approach to each condition as well as the interaction between or among the various conditions. One should not automatically assume that, because a condition is diagnosed on a given axis, by definition it requires drug therapy or psychotherapy. While the clinician has a stronger reason to consider medication for Axis I conditions, psychosocial interventions, including psychotherapy, are usually important for such patients. In addition, a psychodynamic perspective is helpful in dealing with the often conflictual experience of needing to take medication. The clinician who diagnoses a personality disorder will strongly consider the role of psychotherapy or psychoanalysis while being mindful of the evolving literature on the role of medication in this population.

ON PHENOMENOLOGY AND EVIDENCE

Attempting to further advance consideration of the use of medication by psychoanalysts are the contributions of Roose, who, along with his many collaborators, has been an influential thinker within psychoanalysis on the subject of combined treatment (Cabaniss & Roose, 2005; Roose, 1990; Roose & Johannet, 1998). Roose discourages turning to theories of causality or etiology to inform treatment decisions. He suggests a rather strict phenomenological approach whereby the DSM-IV (American Psychiatric Association, 1994) is utilized to make a diagnosis and then clinical decision-making is determined, as much as possible, on evidence-based medical guidelines. He cautions the psychoanalyst against letting his theorizing blind him to alternative treatment perspectives for which evidence exists.

Whatever shortcomings might exist in utilizing this model (Swoiskin, 2001), the focus is on adopting a more scientific and evidence-based approach that would serve pragmatically to improve patient care. Roose is not interested in emphasizing brain-to-mind causality per se; he is trying to ensure adequate treatment for patients in analysis. These contributions serve as another wake-up call to psychoanalysts to consider somatic therapies.

In the last decade or so, evidence-based medicine (EBM), which proposes that clinical practice should be guided by the best possible evidence, has rapidly come to define an optimal standard of care (Deny, 1999). The gold standard for such evidence is the placebo-controlled randomized clinical trial. Evidence supporting the substantial acute and prophylactic effects of lithium carbonate for bipolar disease or the use of antidepressants in melancholia has proved convincing to most clinicians who readily integrate these findings into clinical decision-making. In general, the more robust the scientific evidence for the efficacy of certain treatments is, the more compelled the clinician is to consider those treatments in his treatment algorithm. This also means engaging the patient in the process of informed consent, especially if these treatments are not being pursued (Cabaniss & Roose, 2005).

While we believe that clinicians benefit from turning to the evidence derived from EBM, we are also aware of the risks and limitations of this approach. First, as Gabbard and Freedman (2006) recently pointed out, there are relatively few randomized, controlled trials of psychotherapy and, because of the requirements of manualization and standardization, such studies tend to differ from what goes on in clinical practice. Second, most studies tend to be brief (because of cost and practical considerations) and disorder specific, though patients typically present to clinicians with a more complex set of problems often tied to personality traits (Zimmerman, Chelminski, & Posternak, 2005). Third, the combination treatment trials that do exist mostly involve cognitive–behavioral or interpersonal therapy, making extrapolations for the psychodynamic therapist speculative at best.

Because of these limitations, Gabbard (2005) notes the recent trend toward effectiveness trials that study treatments in a naturalistic setting, forgoing some of the rigors of efficacy trials (placebo control, for example). This kind of research can aid the clinician in answering a question of fundamental importance: Which therapeutic interventions are most helpful for which patient? Silverman (2005) also notes the potential limitations of a too strict adherence to a medical model for evaluating evidence in the clinical situation and reports the formation of a task force of the American Psychological Association to develop evidence-based guidelines for clinicians that will make use of process outcome studies, systematic case studies, and effectiveness studies.

In reviewing the empirical support for combination treatment, Thase (2003) asserts that, besides chronic or recurrent major depression, the evidence for combined treatment is best established for schizophrenia, obsessive–compulsive disorder, and bipolar disorder. He continues:

> There is little evidence that psychotherapy–psychopharmacology combinations should be considered the standard of care for patients with milder depressive and anxiety disorders (the most prevalent conditions for which people seek treatment). The lack of additive effects may justify use of monotherapies first, based on availability and patient preference, with the alternative strategy used in sequence or in combination if necessary. (p. 138)

Hence, while EBM principles may beneficially be applied to some patients, a substantial number of patients will not present a clinical picture that will neatly fit an EBM treatment algorithm. Other considerations must be weighed. For the psychoanalyst, this will typically involve the generation of hypotheses about how psychic conflict has triggered an episode of illness and/or is expressed within the illness itself. When such hypotheses are developed in the evaluation phase, the clinician will consider the potential value of an exploratory treatment. The patient's preference is an important factor, particularly when alternative approaches are reasonable.

However, there will be times when a patient asserts a preference that may appear to the clinician to be suboptimal. In these instances additional psychoeducation may be valuable, but it may also need to be dealt with as a resistance. Among the factors to consider are character issues, intrapsychic conflicts involving the meaning of medication or psychotherapy, and disordered thinking that is related to the acute state of illness. A clinician who is receptive to the usefulness of various modalities of treatment and embraces a complex model of mental functioning is more likely to skillfully walk the line between respecting a patient's preferences while being attentive to potential defensive activity that can undermine optimizing care.

Mr. C, a middle-aged man, was referred by his internist, who was concerned that he was suicidal when he expressed the anxiety of crashing his car into trucks while driving on the highway and then imagining his death. On interview, Mr. C experienced this fantasy as highly disturbing and ego-dystonic. While not phobic about driving, he would display marked anxiety characterized by autonomic symptoms and a fear of losing control. The symptoms were most consistent with situationally bound (cued) panic attacks.

The therapist considered medication for these symptoms and discussed this option with the patient. Given his fears of being out of control, Mr. C preferred talk therapy over the use of medication or the combination, if possible. A dynamic psychotherapy was begun with the following considerations in mind: His capacity to function was not impaired; he did not have comorbid depressive symptoms and denied any suicidal intent; the precipitous onset of the symptoms together with recent and distant traumas noted later suggested a plausible dynamic hypothesis; and he was psychologically minded and motivated to talk.

Mr. C's anxiety began after witnessing a plane crash into the World Trade Center on 9/11. Part of the landing gear was outside his building as he exited. He knew several people who died in the attack. Earlier in his life, he had repeatedly been in the car with his father, who had a serious problem with alcohol. He recalled his father driving while intoxicated and also remembered driving his enraged, bleeding father to an emergency room after he cut himself fighting with Mr. C's mother. Among the various meanings of his symptom were:

- turning passive into active—reliving the trauma of 9/11—by imagining crashing his car into a truck as a plane had crashed into the towers
- identification with the aggressor—the trucks symbolized a threatening father and, by identification, the patient feared being out of control with his anger

A marked diminution of anxiety and an overall increased capacity to be assertive without fearing hurting others resulted from this exploration. For Mr. C, a psychodynamic approach was effective in resolving his anxiety about being out of control. In other patients, medication may be necessary to ease these symptoms. If a fear of medication causing loss of control exists, as it did for Mr. C, this concern may benefit from psychodynamic exploration.

THE DEVELOPMENT OF A COMPREHENSIVE THEORETICAL MODEL

Increasingly, psychoanalysts and psychiatrists recognize the need to consider the interaction between biological and psychological factors in psychiatric disorders. Psychoanalysts will tend to see the continuities between a patient's character and symptomatic states that often benefit from medication. A growing literature within psychiatry similarly supports a shift away from a categorical approach to a dimensional perspective that links personality clusters as *forme frustes* to more serious illness (Siever & Davis, 1991).

For these reasons, a more complex conceptual and philosophical framework of the mind is necessary. To provide that, we turn to a recent contribution of Kendler (2005), who asks two major questions: How are mind and brain (inter) related and how can different explanatory views of mental illness be integrated? His propositions provide the clinician with a nuanced appreciation of complex mind–brain relationships and multiple causality. This is of foundational importance when considering the interaction of psychodynamic psychotherapy and medication. For this reason, we will highlight relevant aspects of his contribution in some detail.

Kendler asserts that Cartesian dualism, falsely dichotomizing mind and brain, must be abandoned. Affirming Damasio's central thesis in *Descartes' Error* (1994), he notes:

> To reject Cartesian dualism (and accept monism, the view that mental and physical processes are both reflections of the same fundamental stuff) means to no longer consider the mental (or functional) to be a fundamentally different thing from the biological (or organic). Rather, the mental and the biological become different ways of viewing and/or different levels of analysis of the mind–brain system. (2005, p. 434)

However, dualistic thinking continues to infiltrate our approach to patients. As alluded to previously, clinicians may see psychiatric illnesses as "biological" and personality disorders as "psychological" (Roose & Johannet, 1998). We will argue that combined treatment, in most cases, benefits from viewing psychological treatments as also biological (Baxter et al., 1992; Kandel, 1979; Mayberg et al., 2002) and biological treatments as affecting the patient psychologically. This is not to say that psychotherapy and medication are the same or biological in the same way. Rather, it invites a more explicit exploration of how, given the fact that these are kinds of biological therapies, different approaches and pathways may be utilized to effect a favorable therapeutic outcome. Abandoning dualism, therefore, creates theoretical space for combined treatment.

Kendler extends his argument by proposing the acceptance of mind-to-brain causality and brain-to-mind causality. Despite the rejection of dualism, a distinction is made between those parts of the brain that are of central importance for mind (higher cortical regions, for example) and other regions that are more essentially bioregulatory (subcortical regions). Causality is a two-way street: Subjective experience (thoughts, feelings, fantasy, psychic conflict) has an impact on brain (and body) functioning and the brain affects subjective experience (mind). Bidirectional causality is helpful when considering combined treatment in that it encourages the clinician to consider both brain-to-mind and mind-to-brain pathways for therapeutic aims. Psychotherapeutic interventions can be viewed as recruiting mind-to-brain pathways and drug therapy as recruiting brain-to-mind pathways. This view of causality illustrates how, while dualism is rejected, there are times when it is useful to conceptualize aspects of brain function as mind. Some phenomena (e.g., intentionality, fantasy) are best thought of in the language of mind, though they require a functioning brain.

Kendler views etiological processes as complex, overdetermined, and nonlinear, at least for major psychiatric illnesses. For example, genetic vulnerability is typically thought of as an "inside-the-skin" pathway. However, research supports the idea that genetic risk can actually gain expression through an "outside-the-skin" pathway. Specifically, genetic risk factors for major depression increase the probability of interpersonal and marital conflicts that are, in themselves, risk factors for major depression.

This kind of research illustrates the false dichotomy often expressed by a patient's query: Is it my genes or the environment? An interactional model—one that acknowledges the complex relationship between environment and constitution—makes it less likely that the clinician will fall prey to oversimplification. While certain conditions have a very large genetic load (for example, the concordance rate for bipolar disorder in monozygotic twins approaches 0.9), what often determines onset of illness is not the presence or absence of a particular set of genes or certain environmental stressors but rather *a genetic or biological vulnerability that is either attenuated or unmasked by a given environmental stress* (Gabbard, 2005; Kandel, 1999; Suomi, 2003).

We suggest that, while Kendler was writing about a philosophical structure for psychiatry, his propositions provide a theoretically robust basis for considering combined treatment. By avoiding reductionism and dualism and by encouraging bidirectional causality and explanatory pluralism, the clinician is equipped to move into the consulting room better able to tolerate complexity and ambiguity and to consider therapeutic interventions through different causal pathways.

INTERACTIONAL MODELS

Having provided a model of mind–brain relations and multiple causality, we proceed to heuristically useful interactional models for combined treatment that, by its very nature, are more complex than the two-illness model. Interaction can be conceptualized in a number of ways. One involves combining treatment—not to treat comorbidity, but rather to treat one condition by utilizing both "top-down" and "bottom-up" approaches.

The top-down pathway emphasizes mind-to-brain causality and a therapeutic approach that involves the mind of the patient who must actively engage his therapist through language, recruiting systems of meaning including wishes, fears, and fantasy. Relatively intact ego functions like working memory, concentration, and impulse control are required for a top-down intervention. On a neuroanatomic level, this approach acts through higher cortical areas and has a *downstream* effect on "lower" levels of brain functioning that are significantly involved in the clinical picture. The top-down pathway involves the patient as agent and implies the acceptance of intentional causality (i.e., the patient has some responsibility for his suffering as opposed to being stricken by illness), even if that causality is on an unconscious basis. Medication treatment is conceptualized as working through a bottom-up approach. In this view, drugs have a primary effect on subcortical areas of the brain that secondarily have an *upstream* effect on higher cortical centers.

With this model, one can visualize certain conditions as being most responsive to one approach or the other or can consider that a simultaneous *two-pronged approach* will be the most effective way to address a problem. The clinician is free to consider combined treatment as reflecting different pathways that can be recruited and then thoughtfully proceed to consider reasonable options with each particular patient. This can also help the clinician to assess the impact of a top-down versus a bottom-up approach. Are separate symptoms of a clinical picture being worked on or are the two approaches addressing the same symptoms through different but overlapping pathways?

Although not described in the top-down, bottom-up models, psychotherapy and medication may each affect both sets of pathways. For many mental disorders, there is a substantial placebo response rate that may act through top-down pathways. Additionally, current psychoanalytic theories emphasize the possible role of noninterpretive mechanisms of therapeutic action, which may affect subcortical areas—a bottom-up pathway.

Current neuroanatomic models of major psychiatric illness—clinical depression and panic disorder—utilize top-down and bottom-up approaches to describe the pathways to illness and health. Gorman, Kent, Sullivan, and Coplan (2000) put forth a neuroanatomic theory of panic disorder that takes into account both subcortical and cortical pathways. The amygdala, which is seen to be a crucial part of the fear network, is inhibited by both SSRIs and benzodiazepines. Bottom-up pathways involve the use of these drugs primarily to affect amygdala functioning and, secondarily, cortical functioning. Cognitive behavioral therapy and, more recently, psychodynamic treatment appear to be effective in treating panic disorder (Milrod et al., 2007); mobilizing systems of meaning and, in psychodynamic treatments, making the unconscious conscious may have a secondary downstream inhibitory effect on the subcortical fear network. Mayberg et al. (1999), Goldapple et al. (2004), and others have provided evidence for the importance of limbic and cortical systems in clinical depression, also affirming differential top-down and bottom-up effects of psychotherapy and medication. The issue of combining treatment to treat anxiety and depressive illness will be dealt with explicitly in chapter 8.

Metaphors: The "Magnet and Metal Filings" and "Resistance and Obstruction"

Metaphors can assist us in conceptualizing complex interactions and developing a framework for thinking about the interrelationship between mind and brain. They also provide patients with a basis for understanding their experience. Gabbard (1992) has suggested one such metaphor: He has likened the tension between psychological and biological causes to the relationship between a magnet and metal filings. This metaphor is meant to convey how a biological diathesis can function as a magnet—an organizer or attractor—for psychic experience; the phenomenological expression of essential conflicts takes shape through the experience of the biological diathesis. However, at times it can be helpful to consider the metaphor in reverse. A primary psychological conflict can function as the magnet activating an otherwise weak biological diathesis (i.e., the metal filings) to gain expression. The resolution of the psychological conflict as magnet then relieves the patient of the biological diathesis that has been unmasked.

Mr. D, a 30-year-old man working as a technician in a radiology department of a hospital, was hospitalized when he relapsed into a mixed bipolar state with psychotic features. On several occasions he ran about the ward naked, experiencing high sexual desire while thinking he was possessed by the devil. He had "visions" that he would be cut up into pieces. He was a virgin who lived at home with his elderly mother; the latter slept in the same room as him, a behavior rationalized out of worry that he would not sleep. He feared that his mother would not let him back into the house because he was evil. A readjustment in his medication (carbarmazepine and olanzapine) brought about a resolution of his psychosis.

In this vignette, the mixed psychotic and affective state is regarded as a biological magnet that organizes the metal filings of core psychological conflicts around separation, sexuality, and punishment in a highly primitive and terrifying way.

Ms. E, a young woman in analysis with a history of low grade depression and generalized anxiety, developed, for the first time, an obsessional symptom while in analysis as she anticipated the analyst's August vacation. The symptom was an ego-dystonic intrusive thought that she had feces in her mouth. Analysis of the symptom within the transference, particularly her feeling of being devalued and worthless because the analyst was going away, rekindling feelings of abandonment when her father left when she was a child, freed her up to express her anger toward the analyst in a way that felt safe, leading to the resolution of the symptom.

In this vignette, the psychic conflict was the magnet, which recruited a weak biological diathesis for obsessive–compulsive disorder. The symptom resolved with analysis.

Often it can be difficult to tell whether biology is the magnet organizing psychology, vice versa, or both. We are left generating hypotheses that we inevitably test in the clinical situation and constantly evaluate the goodness of fit. Probably the most common way this operates is with the patient who presents with significant mood disorder and character pathology (discussed further in chapter 9). The following is an example of hypothesis testing as it relates to a man with ADHD.

A doctoral student in the neurosciences (previously reported in Sandberg, 1998) presented with anxiety and insomnia while pursuing a competitive academic degree and had an impoverished history of intimate relationships. His early history was significant for a frequently absent father who was also less educated. The patient had surgery for an undescended testicle as a young child. The early formulation of an oedipal level conflict manifesting itself as an inhibition gave way to a new formulation when the patient, free associating to his early childhood experience, told the therapist of a previously concealed piece of his early history. He had been formally tested and diagnosed with ADHD in childhood, and this deficit (concealed for narcissistic reasons in the consultation phase) had interfered with his ability to focus on his studies, an area of interest (brain science) no doubt influenced by his awareness of his deficit.

This specific information surfaced while the clinician was exploring a dynamic hypothesis. The patient had been encouraged to free associate to his early experience in school after speaking about missing his father, who was frequently away. A dynamic model had motivated the clinician's inquiry, which then brought up new data that resulted in a reformulation of the case material. What phenomenologically looked like a primary psychological conflict that would benefit from psychotherapy was reassessed and managed with a trial of stimulants that, for this patient, facilitated not only a productive and increasingly efficient way of working but also the time and energy to become romantically involved and subsequently married. In this case, the biological diathesis was the ADHD state (the magnet) around which the psychological "metal filings" of oedipal conflicts revealed itself. The stimulant resolved both states, though another patient with similar symptoms may have required further psychological help.

Wylie and Wylie (1995) introduced another metaphor for conceptualizing the issue of psychological and biological interaction: the notion of "obstruction," as distinct from resistance, to reflect the core constitutional and/or hereditary factors that impede the progress of psychotherapy or psychoanalysis because they must be modified by medication. If the obstruction is not dealt with pharmacologically, the analytic process cannot proceed. They make an explicit suggestion: Therapists need to consider that a clinical situation marked by tenacious resistances may be obstructed by a biologically based disorder that is unmedicated:

> What occurs when the patient inevitably wraps unconscious meaning around the experience of his or her neurobiological factor, is that the nonpsychological factor becomes embedded in the patient's dynamic resistance, and nidus like accrues more defensive strength. It is this nidus which obdurately refuses to yield to analytic efforts, precisely because it is nonpsychological in origin. (p. 191)

The clinician is also at risk for wrapping unconscious meaning around the experience of a neurobiological factor. To use Gabbard's metaphor, this is an example where the metal filings are confused with the magnet because the magnet is not seen as present. Persistent resistance becomes a clue to step back and consider the presence of a second illness that creates an obstruction in the psychotherapeutic process.

BIMODAL RELATEDNESS

The clinician's evaluation of both biological and psychological etiologies of psychiatric illness is experienced internally as an oscillation between different frames of reference that will encourage an interpretive focus that emphasizes the patient's subjectivity or the introduction of medication. Cabaniss (1998) describes this oscillation as "shifting gears" between these different perspectives and evidence. Sandberg (1998) elaborates on the idea of "bimodal relatedness" (Docherty, Marder, Van Kammen, & Siris, 1977), which is the interpersonal manifestation of shifting gears; that is, it expresses the distinction between being with a patient (with what Freud described as free floating attention) and acting on a patient with medication.

Combined treatment, by definition, involves these differing ways of relating. At times, shifting gears will feel comfortable, offering patient and therapist additional therapeutic leverage that works additively or synergistically. At other times, these different treatment approaches may feel contradictory or antagonistic. These tensions will be elaborated throughout this book. Perhaps it is Jackson (1992) who, in an article on the listening healer, has put it most eloquently:

> The place of listening in depth and with empathy is a crucial element in healing. While the emphasis on looking remains significant in the gathering and appraisal of data, at times it threatens to overwhelm the need for an attentive and concerned listener. There appears to be a natural tension between the two modes that has, in modern times, been translated into a tension between a scientific mode of gathering information and a humanistic mode of knowing sufferers. A healer neglects either one at his or her peril—and at the peril of his or her patients. (p. 1632)

CONCLUSION

In this chapter, we have attempted to provide an overview of the essential and complex theoretical issues that relate to combined treatment for the psychodynamic therapist and psychoanalyst. While current trends within psychoanalysis emphasize a relational perspective, man's corporeal nature reasserts itself when the use of medication is considered. We have observed that psychoanalytic theory has its roots in a biological or somatic basis; clinicians of all theoretical persuasions must maintain the legitimacy of this point of view. We have attempted to elucidate various ways in which clinicians can accomplish that.

We have outlined the evolution in theorizing about combined treatment from a rudimentary two-illness model to more complex interactional models. The two-illness model evolved as a response to the growing wealth of knowledge within biological psychiatry that included genetic studies, brain scan data, and drug studies. It also should be seen as a response to an underlying antagonism by many dynamically and analytically oriented clinicians toward the use of medication. As a corrective, particularly within psychoanalysis, it has served its purpose well, as evidenced by the significant number of analytic patients who now receive medication. In addition, there are some patients with severe mental illness who are well managed by thinking of their illness as biologically determined and medication responsive. We also noted that the two-illness perspective, if rigidly held, could create a reductionism of its own.

We observed that another significant trend within psychoanalysis involved utilizing a phenomenological approach based on the DSM-IV (American Psychiatric Association, 1994) and evidence-based medicine, which served to advance the use of medication for patients in analysis. At the same time, the EBM perspective has important limitations, given the fact that patients in clinical practice often present with a constellation of symptoms that are more complex than those researched.

Having described the potential limits of a two-illness model and evidence-based medicine guidelines, we provided a more overarching theory of mind that provides flexibility while addressing greater complexity. An abandonment of mind–brain duality, the avoidance of reductionism (whether biological or mentalist), and the consideration of bidirectional mind and brain causality are all essential aspects of a contemporary view of mind that can accommodate the place for combined treatment. Combined treatment approaches can usefully be conceptualized through "top-down/bottom-up" models and the use of metaphor.

At times, a psychological state will be viewed as triggering a biologically based illness; in other instances, a medication-responsive syndrome will be seen as intensifying psychological conflict. These reflect only two of the numbers of ways to consider interactional dynamics. As the clinician considers these and other possibilities, he tests his hypotheses in his mind and with his patient, making the best use of the various kinds of evidence he has available to him. This process of oscillation among different frames of reference will be illustrated throughout the remainder of the book and is always present when getting started—the focus of chapter 3.

3

Getting Started With Medication

In chapters 1 and 2 we explored models for how therapists could think about patients in combined treatment. Thus, when the patient enters the consulting room, the clinician's evaluation will involve both shifting gears between different perspectives (Cabaniss, 1998) and considering how biological and psychological factors may interact. The clinician is attempting to determine whether the patient will benefit most from psychodynamic psychotherapy or psychoanalysis, some other form of psychotherapy, medication, or a combined treatment. An evaluation of the suitability for psychoanalytic and psychodynamic psychotherapy will not be covered in this book, except insofar as the patient's capacity to engage in insight-oriented psychotherapy may be affected by symptoms that can be eased with medication. Assessment for psychopharmacological interventions will include some form of systematic identification of the presence or absence of symptoms that are part of a variety of disorders (e.g., mood and anxiety disorders) that have been found to be responsive to medication.

In addition to therapists' assessments, patients will often present with an idea or diagnosis of what is wrong with them that they have developed from their own investigations and experience, including reading and advertisements. In current practice it is not unusual for patients to say things like, "I think I have ADD"; "I've had enough therapy. I'm really more interested in medication at this point"; "I saw a commercial and I may be suffering from depression"; "I want therapy and I want to stay away from medications. They're always finding out bad things about them"; or "I read an article about antidepressants that said people may become suicidal if they take them. That sounds pretty scary to me." The patient's hypotheses about symptoms and proposed treatments contain elements of both realistic assessment and fantasies about what is wrong and what will help. These attitudes and beliefs must be taken into account when making recommendations to patients.

Ultimately, the clinician will enter into a dialogue with the patient about what the patient's problems are and whether psychotherapy, medication, or both are indicated. This chapter identifies a series of factors that therapists should consider to determine whether a patient should begin a combined treatment, discusses how to help patients understand the value of having both medication and therapy, and describes how to address certain negative reactions to these recommendations.

THE DECISION TO COMBINE TREATMENTS

For the purposes of this section, it will be assumed that the therapist has already determined that psychodynamic psychotherapy or psychoanalysis is indicated for the patient and a determination needs to be made about whether the patient should also be on medication. As noted earlier, a systematic assessment of symptomatology will guide recommendations about medication. If the patient meets criteria for a medication responsive syndrome, it is important to have a discussion about the possible use of medication for the disorder, even if ultimately a choice is made not to employ it. However, a decision to medicate is not based on phenomenological evaluation alone. Factors to consider include: the degree of the patient's suffering, whether the patient is at risk for self-destructive behavior, and the level of disruption of the patient's functioning. If the patient is beginning psychotherapy, the degree of potential disruption from symptoms, such as difficulties with concentration and motivation, is relevant. Another factor is the patient's preference for treatment, which will be discussed in more depth later.

As described in chapter 2, evidence suggests that a single treatment, either psychotherapy or psychopharmacology, may be all that is needed in many instances. Even when combined treatment is recommended, patients may elect to try one or the other treatment alone initially. In other instances, treatments occur in a sequence; sometimes patients are begun in psychotherapy and subsequently medication is added or psychotherapy added to medication. Each of these is an option, depending on patient preference, responsiveness to the initial treatment, and the developing relationship between patient and therapist.

Mr. F, a 38-year-old man, presented for treatment after becoming increasingly withdrawn from his wife, with whom he had a very limited sexual relationship, and pulled toward involvements with other women that were exciting but not emotionally satisfying. He was fearful of leaving his wife, with whom he still felt emotionally close, and yet was angry at her because he felt there was little excitement in their lives (lack of social activity, shared interests). He became increasingly depressed and presented for consultation with symptoms of major depression.

Mr. F described a background in which, due to his mother's volunteer activities and father's busy work schedule, he received little emotional attention. However, when his mother was at home, he found her to be highly intrusive, with little respect for emotional boundaries. For instance, his mother would press him for details about his social involvements, including his interest in girls. Thus, Mr. F spent significant energy on keeping just the right distance in his relationships. His avoidance of closeness would leave him feeling isolated and alone. He also employed intellectualization and debate to help keep a safe distance.

Although the therapist was concerned that he would be seen as intrusive, like the patient's mother, when exploring Mr. F's inner life, the patient did not appear threatened in this early phase of therapy. He seemed to feel the therapist kept a respectful sense of distance when he indicated that he was getting uncomfortable with a topic. The therapist was aware that he was not pursuing the patient's feelings and fantasies as assertively as he usually would. Notably, however, the patient did appear distressed when the therapist brought up medication.

Mr. F responded that he was unwilling to consider a medication trial.

Therapist: What concerns do you have about medication?

Mr. F: I feel that these drugs aren't safe. They can damage your body.

Therapist: Well, I understand your concerns, but I would like to understand more about what you mean by damage.

Mr. F: I read somewhere that they can affect your liver.

Therapist: In actuality, the antidepressants I am suggesting will not damage your liver or any other organs. Also, depression has been found to potentially harm your body, including over time your heart and immune system. Drugs that help with depression can actually reduce these risks.

Mr. F: You obviously mean well, but you're not the one taking the medication.

Therapist: It sounds like it may be hard for you to trust me on this topic. We do have the option of starting you in therapy alone and seeing how that works.

The therapist recognized a likely link between Mr. F's fears of medication and the feeling of damage caused by his mother's intrusiveness. However, he felt it would be confusing for Mr. F to make this interpretation at this time. He believed it would be better to respond to the patient's concerns with psychoeducation and note that his fears were meaningful and important. They decided to continue the treatment as psychotherapy alone. However, after a few months, as his depressive symptoms persisted despite psychotherapeutic progress, Mr. F agreed to medication. At that point the therapist was able to relate worries about medication to perceptions of his mother in a way that was helpful in relieving his fears.

PATIENT PREFERENCES

When patients express preferences with regard to treatment, these preferences may be based on rational evaluation and choice, a resistance related to patients' conflicts, or both. The therapist may want to explore the patient's choice, especially if the patient is requesting a treatment that the therapist feels is inadequate. For instance, patients who prefer a medication treatment could be basing their request on what they have learned about their symptoms or employing it as a resistance to addressing issues in psychotherapy. The therapist can either accept the patient's choice and evaluate how the patient responds to a medication treatment alone or attempt more actively to address the patient's resistance to a combined treatment.

For instance, Sandberg (1998) describes the case of a patient who presented for treatment after reading *Listening to Prozac* (Kramer, 1993) and specifically requested medication and not psychotherapy to treat his recurrent depressive episodes. In addition to his depressive symptoms, Mr. G reported a feeling of being inauthentic when not depressed. The patient viewed much of his life as a performance, apparently stemming from a mother who had a narcissistic investment in his becoming a successful child actor. Although Sandberg felt this issue should be addressed in psychotherapy, he proceeded as Mr. G had requested, prescribing an antidepressant, to which the patient's symptoms responded. However, Mr. G was disappointed that he was not "transformed" by the medication, as in cases he had read about in Kramer's book.

At that point the patient entered into a psychotherapy, which he experienced as another performance. As the therapist explored Mr. G's sense of inauthenticity and lack of feeling, it emerged that the patient held onto a view that his problems were biological in order to rationalize a feeling of failure in his life. This understanding, along with other developments in the patient's life, allowed him to enter into an intensive psychotherapy, where a strong negative maternal transference could be explored.

PRESCRIBING VERSUS NONPRESCRIBING THERAPISTS

If a decision is made to pursue medication treatment in addition to psychotherapy, the clinician will discuss with the patient whether he will be prescribing it or whether the patient will go to another clinician for additional evaluation and potential medication treatment. A therapist who is a psychiatrist will have the option to medicate the patient, whereas a therapist who is not a psychiatrist will need to send the patient to a psychiatrist for further assessment. At the present time, there is little consensus about whether it is best for the psychiatrist–therapist to refer the patient to a psychopharmacologist or provide both treatments. These issues will be discussed further in chapters 6 and 7.

Patients may react adversely to being sent to another health professional for medication, including reactions such as: "But I want to just see you"; "How come you can't prescribe the medication?" "Are you concerned you cannot handle me?" or "Will I still see you?" Included in these questions is the fear that the therapist may be rejecting them because they are too difficult in some way. Therapists should be alert to these potential reactions and keep them in mind as they explain to the patient the basis for the consultation and how it will work. As usual, positive reactions also occur: "My therapist is willing to accept that I need help that he cannot give me." Further aspects of "treatment triangles" will be discussed in chapter 7.

USE OF THE TWO-ILLNESS VERSUS INTERACTIONAL MODEL

As noted in chapter 2, the model the therapist uses will affect how he thinks about combining treatments and what he communicates to patients. It will often guide how the recommendation for combined treatment is presented. A therapist using a two-illness model might say:

> You have psychological conflicts, but you also have symptoms consistent with a diagnosis of major depression. Therapy will be helpful for your conflicts, but medication will be important for the depression. Treatment of the depression with medication will help you to explore your conflicts.

Alternatively, a therapist employing an interactional model may say:

> You have psychological conflicts and you also have symptoms of major depression. It is likely that your psychological conflicts exacerbate your depressive illness and that your depression adds to your psychological conflicts. Therefore, both treatments would be of value.

In general, we find that use of the interactional model provides patients a better understanding of combining treatments.

Mr. H was in psychotherapy for long-standing feelings of alienation from others, associated with low self-esteem and feelings of inadequacy. He also described chronic fatigue, difficulty concentrating, and pessimism. These symptoms appeared to relate to traumatic events in the patient's past. Specifically, after an extended period of marital discord, his mother moved with Mr. H to another city that had a very different culture. Although she initially told him that his father would be following them there, apparently this was never the plan, and after about a month she told Mr. H that his father was not coming. Mr. H felt alienated in his new environment and had significant trouble adapting. Other children made fun of him due to his different accent and clothes. Subsequently, his mother married a man who was very critical of him, adding to his feelings of distress, inadequacy, and humiliation. In Mr. H's view, his relationships with others never recovered from these early conflicts.

At the time of presentation, Mr. H struggled with social anxiety that inhibited his satisfaction with relationships and his career pursuits. The therapist initially suggested medication for the patient, but Mr. H was against it, feeling that his difficulties were primarily related to problems in his past. In his view, starting medication would minimize the contribution to his problems made by his parents, toward whom he was quite angry. After several psychotherapy visits, the therapist became concerned that Mr. H's problems with energy and concentration were disrupting his treatment.

Therapist: I think you should reconsider medication.

Mr. H: Why is that?

Therapist: These symptoms you describe have really lasted a long time and are making it harder for you to work in therapy. They are symptoms that typically respond to medication.

Mr. H: I'm not really in favor of medication. I think I'm just going to have the same problems to deal with anyway.

Therapist: I know that is part of your usual pessimism, and we have talked about your anger and despair about feeling unable to control what has happened in your life, but pessimism may also be part of your depression. In fact, your low self-esteem, concentration problems, and low energy appear to be part of a syndrome called dysthymic disorder that has been found to be responsive to medication.

Mr. H: I'll consider taking it, but I know there are all kinds of theories about what's wrong. I think it has to do with the anxieties I've had for a long time with people. It comes from my problems with my parents.

Therapist: I certainly agree that we need to talk more about your feelings and early experiences to ultimately help you, but I think part of your symptoms are also biological and would be relieved more quickly with medication. The problems in your early life may have also affected you chemically as well, leading you to be more vulnerable to anxiety and depression. I also think the ongoing stress you have from problems with your relationships may be contributing to your depression and anxiety, making it even harder for you to feel safe with others.

Mr. H: Well I hadn't really thought these experiences might have affected me in a chemical way.

In this case the therapist recognized that Mr. H's anger at his parents added to his being against medication. Thus, he was annoyed by the therapist's comments emphasizing a biological origin of his symptoms, experiencing these as devaluing. This irritation would mirror conflicts he had with his mother, based on the sense that she had misunderstood what he needed and was unresponsive to his concerns. Working with this issue in the transference, however, was difficult to do at this early stage. Mr. H did respond when the therapist used a more interactional model, looking at the way that current and past stresses may have triggered or intensified depressive symptoms.

HOW DO MEDICATION AND PSYCHOTHERAPY WORK TOGETHER?

When patients begin in a combined treatment, they are often curious as to how psychotherapy and medications work together. In these instances, the therapist's understanding of the theories of combined treatment are of value. Patients can be educated about research that suggests that the combination of treatments may be more effective for some disorders. The analyst can explain more specifically how the treatments are synergistic—for example, "medication will help with psychotherapy because you will have more energy and will be able to focus better on what we are discussing." Another comment might be: "Your anxiety is so severe that it disrupts your thinking and makes it difficult for us to explore where it is coming from psychologically."

An additional metaphor to those described in chapter 2, referring to tributaries in a river, can help educate patients about the value of a combination of medication and psychotherapy. In this conceptualization, symptoms are viewed as equivalent to a river flooding its banks. Tributaries to the river include psychological, chemical, and environmental flows. Medication can help to reduce the chemical contribution to the symptoms and psychotherapy diminishes the psychological sources.

Clinicians may be concerned about being too reductionistic in separating biological and psychological aspects of the disorder (the two-illness model discussed in chapter 2). They could add an additional component to the metaphor: Smaller tributaries connect psychological, chemical, and environmental flows, allowing for interaction among the various factors. However, this may make the metaphor too complex for some patients. The clinician could simply state that this model is somewhat oversimplified because psychology, biology, and environment affect each other and each can contribute to the propensity to develop symptoms. Thus, different approaches may aid in relieving patients' distress.

ENCOURAGING PATIENTS TO THINK ABOUT PSYCHOTHERAPEUTIC EXPLORATION ALONGSIDE USE OF MEDICATION

While helping patients to understand why they are in need of medication, the psychodynamic psychotherapist or psychoanalyst also wants to encourage the patient to explore the psychological sources of the disorder.

This not only aids in the development of the analytic process, but also helps to keep the patient from thinking of biology as the only potential source of his problems. Although there are instances in which medication may diminish or avert the need for psychotherapy, in many cases psychological as well as chemical vulnerabilities contribute to the onset of mood disorders and psychotherapy is indicated. It is important for a therapist to help to clarify psychological vulnerabilities, to lay the groundwork for the psychotherapeutic intervention of a proposed combined treatment.

For example, Mr. I explained how he became increasingly depressed after a breakup with his girlfriend and began to get vegetative symptoms and suicidal ideation:

Mr. I: I don't get how I got this depression. I know you think medication would be helpful, but I wouldn't want it to happen again. How do I understand what happened?

Therapist: When you broke up with your girlfriend, you were very upset. But at some point, you became preoccupied with her and you noticed that you couldn't concentrate or sleep well. I believe that this is when you developed a more severe depressive disorder that could respond to medication.

Mr. I: Well, it was very scary. That's when I began having suicidal thoughts. I'll agree to consider medication. What can I do to prevent this in the future?

Therapist: Well, I think it's important to be aware of the recurrence of any of the signs and symptoms that you noticed: reduced energy, insomnia, depressed mood, etc. But I also think it's important that you understand something about the stresses that appeared to trigger this. What was it about this relationship that affected you so greatly? What are you looking for in a relationship and what kinds of problems have you tended to get into? How can you better enjoy your work, which you described as having been increasingly frustrating and meaningless for you? You note that you typically simply accommodate others, and I think this has led to ongoing frustrations for you in your relationships.

Mr. I: Oh yes. That makes sense. I think there are a lot of important things to look into here.

Patients often experience significant relief of their symptoms after medication is started. This improvement will sometimes raise questions in patients' minds as to whether they really need psychotherapy or psychoanalysis. This may lead to further discussion about the potential values of combined treatment.

Mr. J had recently entered treatment that combined medication and psychotherapy. He experienced a fairly rapid resolution of his vegetative symptoms of depression, which he attributed to the impact of medication.

Mr. J: I feel much better now. I'm not really sure I need any more therapy.

Therapist: Well, it's actually not clear which of the treatments is primarily responsible for your improvement at this time.

Mr. J: I know that, but I also had some therapy before and these symptoms did not get better.

Therapist: I can certainly see how you feel at this point. However, I believe that there are certain issues and conflicts that you struggle with that go beyond the impact of medication.

Mr. J: Well, I'm sure everyone has problems. But you know, my job is very busy. It's hard for me to come in for sessions.

Therapist: Yes. I understand that. But you have also spoken about ongoing trust issues with your wife, including concerns that she might have had an affair. And she has said to you that you distance yourself with work.

Mr. J: I agree that there are feelings that are difficult for me to deal with. Do you think the therapy could help me with those problems?

Therapist: Yes. I think we could help you understand the fears you have of getting close to your wife. I mean you have mentioned how difficult your parents' marriage was and how much this affected you.

Mr. J: That's true, although I'm not sure how much that affects me now. But then will I also need the medication?

Therapist: Certainly at first. The medication not only seems to be helping to treat your depression. I think it might also help you to face the fears you have with your wife.

Mr. J: Well, I'm willing to try it.

As with the case of Mr. G, sometimes patients may not be willing to consider pursuing a psychotherapeutic treatment, even after the therapist has explored the value of psychotherapy and patients' resistances to it. In these instances, it makes the most sense to let them continue in medication management alone. If the psychoanalyst is conducting the medication treatment, this can be of value because the analyst can point out, where relevant, what benefits a concurrent psychotherapy might have. In other instances, medications alone can ease personality problems and intrapsychic conflicts, which may have been exacerbated by the psychiatric disorder, and medication alone will be satisfactory.

ASSESSING POSSIBLE REACTIONS BASED ON PERSONALITY FACTORS

Awareness of certain personality factors can help the therapist to predict potential problems that may arise when starting medication and possible approaches to managing these difficulties. Forrest (2004) catalogues a variety of reactions to medication based on characterological predispositions. For instance, obsessional patients may overly focus on specific details of dosing, symptomatic change, and side effects, thus obscuring emotional reactions to the prescribing of medication. Forrest suggests that these patients may also harbor a secret competitiveness with an urge to undermine treatment. Histrionic patients tend to view medications as "magic potions given by their hero, the doctor, to come to their rescue and solve their problems" (p. 367). In these cases, as with narcissistic patients, therapists need to be alert to the disappointment that occurs when the medication does not relieve all distress or side effects become troublesome.

Mr. K, a 54-year-old man, developed the onset of depressive symptoms following retirement from a highly successful career in business. In addition to being depressed, he was bored, and had trouble finding activities that brought him pleasure. He was frustrated by conflicts with his son and daughter-in-law that limited access to his grandchildren. He averred that he had always struggled with feelings of emptiness, relieved only when he had a major success in his career.

Although his depressive symptoms diminished with a combination of sertraline and bupropion, he was frustrated by both sexual side effects and the persistence of his empty feelings. The therapist discussed the fact that, although his lack of pleasure may represent a persistent depressive symptom, it was also possible that medication might not relieve this symptom.

Mr. K continued to press the therapist to give a series of medication trials, while at the same time he admitted he was looking for a "happy pill." He also wanted the "latest" pill that others had not tried, something "special." In this case the therapist continued to work with the patient's preferences, while at the same time emphasizing that the best approach to his symptom might be psychotherapy that looked at the need to feel "special." Ultimately, he returned to sertraline and bupropion and became more willing to engage in psychotherapeutic exploration. However, his ongoing frustration and narcissistic issues limited his involvement with therapy.

INITIAL VERSUS MIDPHASE ADDITION OF MEDICATION

The timing of the addition of medication is relevant to the therapeutic relationship and transference/countertransference issues. The patient who starts medication at the beginning of treatment usually has not developed a significant transference relationship to the therapist. He (or she) may have transference reactions and will likely have positive and/or negative responses to the suggestion of medication. Positive responses include a sense of the therapist competently recognizing his disorder, with an appropriate effort to relieve suffering. Negative fantasies include the notion that the therapist thinks he is too ill for psychotherapy or that the therapist did not understand what he was looking for in treatment.

The therapist should be alert to reactions that he is having to the patient as well and how that might affect the decision to recommend medication.

Suggesting medication is more complex at a later point in the treatment. The therapist should evaluate what transference and countertransference factors may be triggered or affected by the decision. Transferential reactions can include a fear that the therapist is suggesting medication because the patient is unable to tolerate certain wishes or fears that are being dealt with at that time, such as sexual or aggressive fantasies. A patient in the midst of a transference in which he views the therapist as harsh or judgmental may be concerned that the therapist is punishing him. The analyst should consider whether something is emerging that he, the therapist, is having trouble with, such as an intense affect or catastrophic fantasies that the patient has previously felt unable to reveal safely. He should reflect on whether there is a particular transference experience that he is having difficulty tolerating, such as rage and disappointment with the analyst or a demand that the analyst do more to relieve the patient's suffering.

None of these transference/countertransference dynamics indicate that the patient does not need medication. As noted earlier, when a systematic assessment suggests that the patient suffers from a DSM-IV (American Psychiatric Association, 1994) disorder, medication can and should be considered. Transference and countertransference reactions could be painful or negative because patients are having symptoms, caused by biological factors, that the therapy is unable to relieve. Countertransference factors, such as wanting to conduct a "pure" analysis or psychodynamic psychotherapy, could prevent the appropriate use of medication. Concordant transference reactions, such as wanting to please the analyst by not taking medication, could also play a role.

Case Example

Mr. L, a 44-year-old artist, had ongoing concerns that he was suffering from significant depressive symptoms. His therapist had informed him, however, that he felt that medication would interfere with the progress Mr. L was making in psychotherapy. Although Mr. L liked his therapist and believed he had made progress, he felt his therapy had stalled, due in part to difficulty concentrating. Finally, after a prolonged internal struggle, Mr. L went to see a psychopharmacologist without informing his therapist. He experienced a mixture of guilt, frustration, and a fear of disappointing his therapist. In consultation, the psychopharmacologist, who was analytically trained, assessed the patient for medication and also explored his struggle with his therapist. Mr. L was perceiving the analyst as his terrifying and otherwise unresponsive father. He typically needed to go behind his father's back to get comfort from his mother, who both submitted to and rebelled against her husband's demands. The patient also clearly described significant depressive symptoms, and a medication trial was in order. The psychopharmacologist was able to convince Mr. L to talk to his therapist about having obtained the consultation. He also, with the patient's agreement, contacted the therapist and helped to educate him about the role of medication in this instance.

The therapist had been aware of some frustration with Mr. L's apparent "resistance," but was interested to learn that depressive symptoms may have been contributory. With this new information, the therapist was able to reconceptualize the patient's efforts to obtain medication as not simply "acting out" and explored with Mr. L why he felt he needed to go to the psychopharmacologist without letting him know. He acknowledged to Mr. L that he had in fact underestimated the need for medication. Rather than this being a basis for terminating the discussion of this topic, the therapist and patient productively explored how the developments in therapy related to the patient's early experience.

Although this case describes factors involved in a "treatment triangle," a topic that will be covered in chapter 7, in this instance it demonstrates complex transference/countertransference feelings and fantasies that can surround the consideration of medication at a midphase point. Appropriate consideration of the issues can help to minimize potential disruptions in treatment, and proper attention can allow these dynamics to be employed to further the therapy. In this case, progress was made with the relief of depressive symptoms and the elaboration of the conflicts that psychologically inhibited Mr. L's assertiveness in a number of situations.

HUMILIATION ABOUT MEDICATION

Many patients will experience the need for medication as evidence that they are sick and weak in some way. This issue is important to address in terms of its impact on self-esteem, its meaning, and the potential disruption in compliance. In particular, patients seeking psychodynamic psychotherapy may not have grappled with the notion that medication may be in order. They may hear a psychoanalyst's recommendation for medication as a suggestion that they are "too ill" for therapy alone. A different problem may emerge at midphase, at which point patients may feel the therapist is no longer able to tolerate the particular symptoms, conflicts, or transference fantasies occurring at that time, adding to feelings of shame about what they are experiencing.

Ms. M described a long history of focusing on her ears, which she viewed as rendering her unattractive and of little interest to men. It emerged that her family was very concerned about appearance and, to some degree, she was dismissed by her father's family as not being attractive enough. In reality, the patient received a great deal of positive feedback from men. Nevertheless, a sense of her being defective would intermittently become prominent, creating a depressive and anxious state. When medication was discussed during the initial consultation, Ms. M was very distressed, in spite of her agreement to start it. Even as the patient was experiencing significant relief of her symptoms, it emerged that she felt humiliated about needing to take it.

Therapist: What troubles you about being on the medication?

Ms. M: Well, I feel defective. It means something is terribly wrong with me. You don't think therapy is enough for me.

Therapist: That sounds a lot like how you feel about your ears and your family's reaction to your appearance.

Ms. M: Yes. I guess it does, but I'm worried that you see me in that way. How do you explain my need for medication?

Therapist: It sounds like you feel I'm going to react to you as your father did: that I will reject you because of something "wrong" with you. I certainly do not see the use of medication as a sign of a defect, but I do think it will ease your level of distress and help us to understand better what is causing your feelings of shame.

Ms. M: Well, it doesn't feel like you're behaving like my father. He would really criticize me if I brought up my concerns with him. I guess I must have felt that having any kind of problems meant I was bad.

In this case the therapist was able to use a basic understanding of the patient's history, developmental conflicts, and early transference reactions to help her gain some understanding of what was troubling her about medication. The vignette also indicates how combined treatments can work synergistically. Noncompliance with medication is an important clinical problem, and humiliation about taking medication is one factor that disrupts compliance. Being able to help relieve patients of these negative feelings therefore can aid in their continuing medication. Once medication is effective, it can diminish feelings of humiliation that are part of the depressive disorder.

As noted previously, suggesting medication at midphase presents problems more closely related to the active transference/countertransference dynamics. In the following case, painful feelings emerged in the transference when the subject of medication was discussed after the patient reported depressive symptoms and suicidal ideation. Ms. N's father was a doctor whom she experienced as critical and disconnected from her needs. She tended to see doctors in general as potentially hurtful individuals from whom she had to protect herself.

Ms. N: I feel that I made too big of a deal about how upset I was, that I was thinking about taking my own life. Now you think I'm crazy and in need of medication. I behaved like a drama queen. I just need to get hold of myself.

Therapist: I'm not sure what you mean when you say I think you're crazy.

Ms. N: That you think I'm weak and that there is something wrong with me. I wasn't able to respond to therapy.

Therapist: This sounds a lot like how you'd view your father's thoughts about you.

Ms. N: Well, that's true. He always was very critical of me. But now I'm being told something is very wrong with me.

Therapist: Well, I guess I don't really think about it in those terms. I certainly think you have depression and that it is greatly increasing your suffering. I don't really view that in the category of weakness. I think we need to understand why you feel so self-critical about it.

Despite these discussions of the patient's concerns, Ms. N remained unwilling to take medication. Because he was somewhat concerned about the patient's safety, the therapist increased his efforts to get Ms. N to begin the medication, elaborating on the symptoms it would treat and warning of the risks of not taking it. At this point, the therapist became aware of having entered into an enactment with the patient in which he was behaving like the patient's father, with whom she struggled for control. The therapist described this dynamic to the patient and, being aware of it, they were able to move away from these positions and cooperatively explore the value of medication.

THE ANALYST'S STANCE

A major potential problem in integrating combined treatment derives from the different orientation and technique of these two approaches. Psychopharmacological treatment tends to focus on systematic assessment of symptoms, dosages, and side effects, and the treating psychiatrist is directive and prescriptive. The analytic model calls for an open-ended, free associative interaction in which the analyst comments on the patient's productions. Although this is less of a problem when the analyst is not prescribing, the therapist should still be alert to the presence of symptoms, the impact of medication, and medication side effects because these will invariably weave into the content of treatment.

Kelly (1998) described two views of the psychoanalyst treating a patient with medication: the "abstinent" and the "interventionist" models. According to the abstinent model, a psychoanalyst prescribing medication violates the principles of abstinence and neutrality because he becomes involved with the patient in a nonanalytic mode. Even if it is helpful to the patient, it disrupts the therapist's ability to function analytically, and therefore the analyst should avoid prescribing or being in close contact with the psychopharmacologist. The alternate perspective derives from the interventionist model, in which the analyst prescribes the medication.

Kelly argues that the interventionist model should be used only if the analyst maintains an appropriate degree of neutrality. Cases that allow this approach, in his view, are those in which medical management is not likely to be complicated, medication is not essential so that the analyst can respond neutrally to the patient's decision about taking it, and the pleasurable or unpleasurable effects of the medication are not immediate.

However, Kelly's description confuses technical neutrality (being equidistant from id, ego, and superego) with the analyst being neutral about whether or not the patient takes medication. This misunderstanding disrupts the analyst's ability to appropriately address the patient's status with medication. The analyst may withhold a recommendation of medication or feel inhibited to address side effects, due to a perceived need to remain neutral. In addition, it is unclear that the analyst's ability to analyze is disrupted by these interventions. Thus, the analyst pursuing medication treatment of the patient's illness need not feel he has breached an essential analytic attitude.

Concerns about a prescribing stance are less common in the initial evaluation period, when the typical approach is semistructured and information gathering, aimed at understanding the psychological and neurophysiological contributors to symptoms. When medication intervention occurs at midphase, however, the therapist will typically shift from the analytic mode to a semistructured and more directive stance, including psychoeducation about medication, potential side effects, and the hoped-for outcome. Analysts should be alert to their own shift in approach and the potential reaction of the patient. As described earlier, the analyst may not feel comfortable veering away from analytic interventions and may present inadequate information or, alternatively, become overly rigid and directive. Patients could feel demeaned or distanced by the analyst's shift, experiencing it as a move away from the treatment as collegial investigators of the patient's psyche or relieved by the "break" from analytic exploration.

Ms. M, described previously, became upset when the therapist discussed the dosing of her antidepressant medication, which was being restarted later in her therapy after a recurrence of depression following pregnancy. The therapist was somewhat puzzled by her reaction because he and the patient had had several discussions regarding the value of the medication, and the patient was now in full agreement with the plan.

Therapist: You seemed upset just now when I started talking about the doses of the medication.

Ms. M: Yes. You seemed more distant.

Therapist: Can you say more?

Ms. M: I'm not sure, but all of a sudden it felt like you were the doctor and I was the patient, and somehow you were better than me. You're not usually like that.

Therapist: Do you think I actually changed my attitude or is that how it felt?

Ms. M: I'm not really sure.

Therapist: Well, it certainly sounds like how you described your home, with you being told what to do and very little being discussed with you.

Ms. M: Yes, and that somehow you're just better than me. I mean I guess you really weren't acting that way.

The therapist, after reflecting on the patient's comments, realized that his stance was somewhat different when discussing the medication and that his tone probably sounded more authoritative. The patient experienced this as being demeaned, as she felt in her own home when she was often criticized by her father for not understanding something he said or debating ideas with him. The analyst's psychopharmacological stance triggered this transference reaction, which was productively explored.

Although the analyst's stance is different in assessing and prescribing medication in comparison to that in psychoanalysis, efforts can be made to minimize the discrepancy. As noted previously, the therapist should be making a recommendation but also encouraging the patient to think about the medication intervention and the impact of the medication psychologically. How does the patient feel about taking the medication? What are the patient's concerns? Another part of this process is engaging the patient in thinking about how medication is affecting his fantasies, conflicts, and levels of anxiety and depression, as well as his experience of the analyst. These inquiries will convey the notion that although the analyst is recommending and/or prescribing the medication, he continues to be curious about the patient's intrapsychic reactions. Explorations of the meaning of medication will be discussed in depth in chapter 4.

A potential interfering factor to exploring reactions to medication is that the analyst (and patient) may consciously or unconsciously want to separate the therapy from discussions about medication. The conceptualization may be: "Now I am being the doctor and talking about medication, and then I will return to being the therapist and deal with the psychological issues." The nonprescribing analyst may think: "I am not involved in medication treatment; I'll refer this matter to the psychopharmacologist." These manifestations of the two-illness model can lead to the therapist ignoring signs and signals he would usually attend to, such as the patient's anxieties and frustrations about the experience of side effects and reactions to the analyst's role in prescribing or cooperating with the physician who is prescribing. As the patient is started on medication, it is important for the therapist to be alert to tendencies to exclude medication from the therapeutic process.

CONCLUSION

During the initial consultation, therapists will identify certain patients as likely to benefit from both psychotherapy and medication. In this diagnostic process, therapists will be applying the two-illness and interactional models and make use of "shifting gears" in their assessment and their discussion of their recommendations with the patient. Therapists should make efforts to foster a developing analytic process and appropriately educate patients about medication. Alertness to patients' reactions to medication, both negative (e.g., humiliation, rejection) and positive (feeling the therapist recognizes their distress), will aid therapists in successfully establishing a combined treatment. Introducing medication at midphase adds additional complexity because therapists must consider active transference and countertransference paradigms, as well as the impact of the shift in their usual psychotherapeutic stance. Whenever medication is started, efforts should be made to include reactions to and meanings of medication in the psychotherapeutic process.

4

The Meaning of Medication

An analytic attitude is characterized by a consistent interest in exploring a patient's inner life and uncovering meaning. From this vantage point, the introduction of medication creates opportunities for deepening analysis and increasing a patient's self-understanding. Patients' anxieties and wishes will be evoked around the introduction and use of medication. As observed in chapter 3, exploring the meaning of medication at the outset of treatment often creates opportunities to engage the patient psychotherapeutically while managing resistance to a pharmacologic intervention.

The introduction of medication during an analysis or psychotherapy will often be experienced through the predominant transference operating at the time; its use can also stimulate new and surprising transferences. Meaning is dynamic and will often change during the course of treatment (Milrod & Busch, 1998; Schlierf, 1983; Tutter, 2006). For some patients, the importance of medicine lies in the way it is used to impede a deepening introspective process. Medication can serve as a vehicle for enactments, the analysis of which can advance the treatment (Abel-Horowitz, 1998). At other times, the insistence on exploring the meaning of medication can reflect the presence of countertransference (Awad, 2001).

In this chapter, we will explore these issues with the following questions in mind:

What are the countertransference reactions that can interfere with the exploration of meaning?

How do cultural factors influence the meaning that patient and analyst attach to medication?

How does the analyst think about the placebo effect and when is it explored?

What is the nocebo effect and what are its manifestations?

How does one approach medication use as a transitional object?
What other manifestations of pill as object exist?
What are some of the ways in which transference and countertransference are elaborated around the use of medication?
When is the exploration of meaning a manifestation of countertransference?

COUNTERTRANSFERENCE IMPEDIMENTS TO THE EXPLORATION OF MEANING

A number of factors can adversely affect a therapist's openness to exploring the meaning of medication with a patient. Witness the fact that while approximately 30% of analytic patients receive medication, there is a paucity of papers in the literature on the topic. Gwynn and Roose (2004) report that, among candidates in training, little if any reference to medication exists in their writing about the psychoanalytic process. Because these candidates are being taught and supervised by experienced analysts, these findings suggest a pervasive countertransference problem. This is particularly striking because the study took place at the Columbia Center for Psychoanalytic Training and Research, where significant work on combined treatment has taken place. An awareness of some of the common factors that can interfere with analytic curiosity about medicine can help the clinician avoid such pitfalls.

Chapter 1 outlined some of the early resistances to the use of medication, and chapter 3 explored these issues as they affect starting medication. We suggest that the reluctance to explore the meaning of medication is derivative of these early conflicts. The importance of technical purity with its emphasis on the mutative power of interpretation placed pharmacotherapy outside the bounds of preferred technique. Some authors have suggested that "parameter" is a useful term for the introduction of medication into an analytic treatment (Kelly, 1998); others have recommended abandoning it because of a negative connotation that discourages the use of drugs and other noninterpretive interventions (Awad, 2001). Is the clinician aided or burdened by thinking of medication use in this way?

Eissler (1953) introduced the term to refer to a deviation from abstinence and neutrality—one intentionally undertaken by the analyst because the patient's condition required more active intervention. Parameters were to be used only if necessary and as long as their significance could be explored. Some therapists of the relational school would reject outright the importance, if not plausibility, of abstinence and neutrality as analytic ideals. Others, coming from an ego psychological or object relations perspective, would continue to see these as useful clinical guideposts for technique while appreciating the importance of the psychotherapeutic relationship as a two-person psychology. This viewpoint includes the inevitability of enactments as vehicles for analytic exploration and the real person of the analyst as an essential aspect of the clinical endeavor. While these shifts within contemporary psychoanalytic theory and practice have contributed to a widening scope within the discipline, there is an enduring ambivalence on the part of many analysts to meld the *pure gold* of analysis with the use of medication (e.g, see Caligor et al., 2003). We believe, in agreement with Awad (2001), that the use of the term "parameter" risks perpetuating, however inadvertently, the stigmatization of both medicine and analysts who make use of it in their practices. The analyst can feel that medication represents a second-rate treatment (Roose & Johannet, 1998).

The devaluation of medication as a therapeutic tool can create a ripple effect where the patient is devalued for not being an "ideal" patient, and the analyst feels devalued for not being an "ideal" analyst. To bolster his or her analytic sense of self, the therapist can proceed by turning away from medication-related issues. Candidates are particularly vulnerable, as they are in an early stage of identity formation as analysts. We suspect this is one reason they tend to exclude references to medication in their write-ups as described previously (Gwynn & Roose, 2004). Rather than viewing treatment integration as an expression of an analytic sensibility, the idea is expressed—overtly or covertly—that medication is irrelevant or secondary.

Countertransference issues can also be evoked when the prescribing therapist feels guilty for creating problematic side effects for the patient (Glick & Roose, 2006). The therapist can be vulnerable to acting to undo the damage (i.e., suggesting a medication change) without exploring the transference implications of the adverse effect. This will be discussed in more detail in chapter 6.

Another manifestation of negative attitudes toward medication can occur in a split treatment when the therapist adopts the attitude that all medication-related phenomena are the responsibility of the pharmacotherapist. Unless the lay therapist has a good familiarity with common therapeutic and side effect profiles, he will not be equipped to deal with them when they surface as part of the patient's free associations. Wylie and Wylie (1996) describe how a patient's rapid response to fluoxetine (within a couple of days) was taken, at face value, as drug response and only later understood as a reflection of a complaint of the slow pace of analysis. If the therapist is not aware that an antidepressant response evolves over weeks, not days, he will not be in a good position to search for the importance of the rapid response. The particular challenges of exploring the meaning of medication in a split treatment will be taken up in chapter 7.

CULTURAL MEANING

Just as the awareness of countertransference vulnerabilities aids the clinician, being attuned to cultural trends also helps. These trends shape and are shaped by the individuals within the culture. While the clinician will be interested in the particular meaning with which a patient invests medication, such meaning unfolds in ways that are either reinforced or discouraged by the culture at large. We focus on Western culture—in particular, the United States. (The interested reader is referred to Elliot & Chambers, 2004, for an enlightening discussion of the contrast between Western and Japanese culture.)

In the United States, a variety of factors have contributed to the popularization of psychotropic medication over the last two decades. Evidence-based medicine, as discussed in chapter 2, reflects a growing trend within general medicine and psychiatry and is most easily applied to medication trials. The introduction of managed care has impinged upon the availability of psychotherapy for many patients who often have to do battle with their insurer or accept significant out-of-pocket expenses. Metzl and Riba (2003) describe the impact of the Food and Drug Administration relaxing regulations on drug companies and permitting direct-to-consumer advertising. This type of advertising, especially for antidepressants, often makes explicit their value to correct a "chemical imbalance." These factors contribute to some patients presenting not only with a specific preference for pharmacotherapy over psychotherapy but also with a particular drug preference in mind.

Nothing captures the current cultural zeitgeist more vividly than the popularity of books written about fluoxetine. In *Listening to Prozac*, Kramer (1993) coined the term *cosmetic psychopharmacology* to describe a clinical response as "better than well." He found that patients with chronic low self-esteem, worry, and anhedonia experienced a profound change in their sense of self after being medicated with fluoxetine. He surmised that these patients suffered from *forme frustes* of anxiety and depressive illness. His clinical descriptions were of patients who seemed neurotic and masochistic. However infrequent this kind of transformational experience may be, fluoxetine and other SSRIs have taken on the status of enhancement technologies (Elliot & Chambers, 2004). Some individuals will be excited by this prospect, others threatened. The cultural manifestation of this ambivalence can be seen in books, such as *Prozac Nation* (Wurtzel, 1995), that strike a cautionary note about its use.

The introduction of SSRIs, a class of drugs that is safer to use than the older tricyclic antidepressants and monoamine oxidase inhibitors, has served to diminish the stigma of mental illness while cultivating an illusion of medication as panacea. The widening scope of pharmacotherapy (with the SSRIs) now includes major depression, dysthymia, panic disorder, obsessive–compulsive disorder, post-traumatic stress disorder, social phobia, premenstrual syndrome, and impulsive aggression in personality disorders. This shift in thinking about medication has coincided with marked advances in technology and an emphasis on increased efficiency. Fluoxetine and other SSRIs, within American culture, seemed to reflect another advance in this direction.

Cultural determinants are the most superficial layer of meaning, though not of superficial importance. A clinician's awareness of these factors will heighten his capacity to empathize with a patient who presents with a strong preference for a particular therapeutic intervention. For many patients it is crucial to explore the fantasies behind their request but also the cultural basis—that is, the external reality—upon which the fantasy has grown. Often patients display an underlying fear of what is inside them and a preference to "medicalize" their suffering. In that way, they align with one facet of the cultural zeitgeist.

THE PLACEBO EFFECT

How does the psychodynamic therapist or psychoanalyst approach the placebo effect? While it varies across different conditions (relatively high in depression and panic disorder while low in mania and OCD), the pharmacotherapist makes use of the placebo effect to encourage a positive outcome of a medication trial. He tries to be hopeful, optimistic, and encouraging, using his benevolent authority to cultivate a positive attitude in his patient. This attitude may be expressed largely through implicit channels of communication—not so much by what is said but by the manner of speaking. In other words, the prescriber's non-neutral attitude likely comprises one facet of the placebo effect. The desire on the part of the patient to be pleased contributes to the therapeutic power of the intervention.

Yet psychoanalysts are trained to be on guard against unduly influencing their patients. An analytic attitude would seem to mitigate against encouraging a placebo response. How does the clinician move between deepening a patient's awareness of his inner life while cultivating through benevolent authority a positive response to a medication trial? These issues will be of particular relevance to the prescribing therapist; however, they also operate in a more subtle way for the therapist whose patient is being medicated as part of a split treatment. The nonprescribing therapist will convey explicitly or implicitly attitudes about the medication that will either encourage or discourage a favorable response. What clinical guideposts can assist him or her?

Contemporary analytic work has moved beyond the more austere, detached, one-person model to one that focuses on the inevitable oscillation between one- and two-person psychologies (Gabbard, 2000). Even among more classically trained ego psychologists, the importance of the real person of the analyst and enactments has been described (Jacobs, 2001). Furthermore, it is an oversimplification to distinguish the prescriber's non-neutral attitude and the investigatory neutrality of the analytic attitude. Benign transference inheres in the analyst's caring role and so can be seen to cover both treatment postures. If medication is indicated, we suggest that the therapist feel free to express a degree of optimism about its use that characterizes the average expectable effect of the drug without being overly zealous or blandly neutral.

Strong reactions in either direction can be a signal of countertransference. The patient needs to process not only the recommendation for medication, but also the therapist's genuine belief that it will help. This posture is appropriate whether the analyst is prescribing or having a colleague assume that responsibility. The technical question involves when to make this interaction the focus of therapy. We suggest the following guidelines:

- The less intensive and more supportive the treatment is, the more likely it is that the placebo effect will be cultivated and left unanalyzed. There will not be sufficient gain to warrant an exploration of what can be conceptualized as a nonobjectionable aspect of the positive transference. The physician gratifies in the act of giving, and the patient is gratified in receiving. In these clinical situations the primary importance of the placebo effect is that it serves to encourage a good therapeutic response to an active drug. Positive references to the medicine, if they are not deemed defensive in nature, are accepted at face value.
- The more intensive the treatment is, the more curious the therapist will be about all aspects of his patient's experience of the medicine, including those particular meanings with which it had been imbued based on the positive transference. Psychoanalysis, in particular, is a treatment where exploring positive aspects of the meaning of medication is likely to surface, given the pivotal work in the transference. These explorations are intended to deepen the analysis. An analyst who recommends medication, whether he is prescribing it or not, will anticipate this action influencing the transference and explore its meaning with the patient.

THE NOCEBO EFFECT: WORKING WITH RESISTANCE

Barsky, Saintfort, Rogers, and Borus (2002) point out that the term *nocebo* (meaning in Latin "I will harm") was originally coined to distinguish the disturbing effects of a placebo from its beneficial, therapeutic effects. Writing about meaning and medication in the treatment-resistant patient, Mintz (2002) observes the high frequency with which "refractoriness," when analyzed, reveals an underlying expectation of harm. This nocebo effect can present as the refusal to accept medication or the experience, often repetitive, of extreme sensitivity to side effects of any medications used. Unlike true refractoriness, these patients seldom tolerate adequate medication trials.

Sometimes it is difficult to differentiate a nocebo effect from problematic side effects; the latter can exacerbate an otherwise mild tendency to experience harm. Whereas the indications for exploring the particular meaning of a placebo effect exist on a continuum, the nocebo effect, especially if repetitive, is an indication for exploratory work. It suggests the presence of an intrapsychic conflict that may need to be resolved as a precondition for an adequate medication trial. For the psychodynamic clinician, the nocebo effect is viewed as resistance, the understanding of which will typically involve work in the transference.

The Nocebo Effect Presenting as Noncompliance

When a medication trial together with psychotherapy was recommended to Mr. O for long-standing symptoms of depression (dysthymia and recurrent major depression) and anxiety (panic disorder, hypochondriasis, and obsessive–compulsive disorder) that had responded incompletely to psychotherapy alone, he insisted that he would be unwilling to swallow a pill to help heal his mind. He was certain that doing so would only worsen his already intolerable anxiety, as he likened the prospect to "fucking with [his] mind." When asked to associate to these concerns, he spoke of a highly conflicted relationship with his father, who often suggested to the patient that he had not sufficiently resolved his emotional problems. The father was experienced as intrusive, controlling, and emasculating. The patient felt castrated by his father—hence passive and receptive—and simultaneously wished to feel loved by him, expressed by the intolerable fantasy of being fucked. The pill had come to represent the father's phallus as a "mind fuck."

Elaborating the negative paternal transference brought the patient more in touch with his sexual frustration with his wife and the terror of his anger. The latter was another determinant of his anxiety in the transference: the projection of his anger onto the therapist so that the therapist's potency as symbolized by the pill was experienced as destructive. Another aspect of his difficulty taking medication, less conspicuous than the paternal transference, was the maternal transference.

The patient had few if any memories of his mother from when he was growing up. He imagined that she had been quite depressed (something she later verified) when he was young. His sense of deprivation heightened his passive yearning for love and nurturance, which fueled intense fears of being helpless and out of control. Over a period of 2 months, the negative transference was analyzed with particular relevance to its manifestation as a resistance to medication. This therapeutic work freed him to accept a sertraline trial because his anxiety diminished. He fleetingly had an upsurge in anxiety with the first low dose of sertraline and then progressively was able to move to a therapeutic dose with a marked reduction in his symptoms. His improvement simultaneously laid the groundwork for further psychotherapeutic work.

For Mr. O, medication had multiple meanings that were open to interpretation. The *act* of receiving medication represented a penetration that had to be fended off. The medication was the phallus, stemming from a paternal transference. The *act* also represented a frightening passivity and helplessness based on yearnings for his mother's love. In this instance, the *medication* was the breast. Mr. O's conflicts over his libidinal and aggressive strivings were apparent in his attitude about medicine and largely manageable by the therapist without the incursion of countertransference. While this largely interpretive approach works for many patients, at other times it is through the evocation of a countertransference reaction that the groundwork for interpretation is laid.

Mr. P presented for a second opinion about his treatment in the setting of multiple medical problems, including recent coronary bypass surgery. He was in a mixed affective state characterized by irritability and agitation while simultaneously slowed down with impaired cognition. He had a severe sleep disturbance and panic attacks which, on more than one occasion, brought him to an emergency room fearing a heart attack. His underlying mistrust of physicians was apparent when, upon presentation, he complained bitterly about his psychiatrist who, according to the patient, charged exorbitant fees and spent little time with him. He subsequently complained that the initial meeting with the consultant had been a waste of time because he had done most of the talking. He had a long history of feeling insecure about his manliness and a capacity to spend money he did not have. His spending was not driven by euphoric periods of mania. Rather, he felt compelled to impoverish himself at the expense of making sure each of his children's every need was met. This left him with a sizeable debt. The diagnostic impression was of a mixed affective state with narcissistic, paranoid, and masochistic character traits.

Initial efforts to control his agitation and sleep with medication had little effect or created a paradoxical worsening of his symptoms. Mr. P repeatedly expressed concerns that medication would damage him despite reassurances to the contrary. In his effort to seize control, he would either take medicine at a lower dose than suggested or take higher doses because he felt "desperate" to feel better. He would then complain that the therapist was of no use to him. After a while, the therapist realized that Mr. P did with verbal interventions what he did with medicine: He seemed unable to accept anything that was given to him without experiencing it as toxic or useless. This left the therapist feeling weak and powerless, an emotional state that resembled that of the patient. This countertransference awareness led the therapist to explore the patient's persistent sense of powerlessness in relation to a caregiver.

Therapist: It's hard for you to depend upon me.

Mr. P: Nothing you're giving me is helping!

Therapist: But you've not given any of the medicines I've given you a fair chance. You either reject them outright or do your own prescribing.

Mr. P: My mother always said the world is filled with two types of people. There are "givers" and "takers." You're like all the other doctors—only interested in taking my money.

Therapist: That's a very black-and-white way to see the world. How do you see yourself?

Mr. P: Definitely a giver! Look at how I've given to my children—at my own expense!

Therapist: Yes, at your own expense. You've not been able to balance taking care of yourself, including being taken care of, with taking care of others. I take your money because this is my livelihood; but that leaves you suspecting my motives as a healer. It's as if I can't give to you because I take. And it's as if you can't take anything meaningful from me because you're so invested in seeing yourself as a giver.

Mr. P: I'm embarrassed to say that if you charged me nothing I think I would be able to trust you. But that's not being fair to you and, I guess, I'm not being fair to myself either. I know I need your help. I can't do this by myself ... or by continuing to fight with you.

Mr. P eventually agreed to a trial of lithium carbonate—something he had initially rejected outright as "poison"—and had excellent mood stabilization. This set the stage for a productive period of psychotherapeutic work.

These examples serve to illustrate how the exploration of meaning unfolds within the transference. LaFarge (2000) has made a useful distinction between the analyst's functioning in an interpretive as opposed to containing mode. The former, illustrated with Mr. O, primarily involves language and interpreting unconscious fantasy. The latter, characterized by Mr. P, often involves the evocation of countertransference feelings within the analyst that form the basis of interpretation. As with other clinical material, the analyst will at times discover meaning through a predominantly interpretive route; at other times, he will utilize his internal reactions to help formulate an interpretation.

The Nocebo Effect Presenting as Pseudocompliance

Sometimes patients manage the nocebo effect by idealizing psychotherapy to compensate for the narcissistic injury of needing medication. Rather than reject the use of medication, this idealization expresses the hope that psychotherapy will obviate the need for medication at some point in the future. The patient displays a split transference: a positive transference toward the clinician as psychotherapist and a negative transference (masked by compliance) toward him as pharmacotherapist. The idealization of the therapist's skills can be particularly seductive and lead the therapist to avoid addressing the patient's ambivalence about needing medication. Such a patient can present highly motivated to engage in verbal therapy as prophylaxis against future episodes of illness, "guaranteeing" a return to a drug-free state.

Mr. Q entered analysis after being seen in consultation and receiving acute treatment for a second episode of major depression some months after he married and his mother committed suicide. He was a soft-spoken, narcissistic man with a thick obsessional veneer. Coming from a culture that supported analysis, he enthusiastically embraced the recommendation when it became clear that significant character issues interfered with his capacity for intimacy. He also raised the idea that analysis would immunize him against further episodes of depression, and this wish motivated him to seek an intensive treatment.

While the analyst observed a psychological trigger for his depressive episodes—namely, an effort to get close to a woman and "make roots"—he also needed to explore the patient's wishful fantasy that analysis would prevent future episodes, a possibility that could not be guaranteed. Rather than threaten his entry into analysis, this exploration permitted the analyst and patient to see how terrified he was of ending up like his mother. Medication, which had failed to help his mother, fueled a frightening identification with her. It reflected not only a severe illness, but also a terminal one.

The Nocebo Effect Due to Change From Medication

The experience of medication as a threat is not confined to the beginning of treatment. Whereas the anxieties around initiating medication permit the therapist to see what the patient has projected onto (or into) it as a kind of Rorschach, the experience of feeling threatened can surface after the medication has been introduced. Paradoxically, the threat can be a reaction to a perceived benefit from the drug. Sometimes this response derives from narcissistic issues that may or may not be amenable to psychotherapeutic intervention.

Dr. R presented severely depressed with suicidal ideation, an inability to function, and quasi-nihilistic delusions. Aggressive psychopharmacology that included the use of an atypical antipsychotic (quetiapine) and mood stabilizer (lamotrigine) brought about a remission of these symptoms, and he gradually returned to work. Premorbidly, he described functioning chronically on a hypomanic level. He typically got by on little sleep, had high self-esteem, and was artistic. Twice divorced, he tended to move around in an impulsive manner that gave his life a quality of uprootedness. The working diagnosis was bipolar type II—periods of hypomania alternating with major depression.

Some months after he had returned to work, Dr. R told his therapist he had stopped all of his medication because he feared it would interfere with his capacity to function. He viewed his therapist's lack of awareness of his noncompliance as evidence that he did not need the medication. Moreover, his creativity as an artist had returned, and he enjoyed sustained periods of productivity while receiving accolades from other artists.

Over a period of months the risks and benefits of preventive treatment with a mood stabilizer were discussed. Prophylaxis was strongly indicated since the patient suffered from years of untreated bipolar spectrum illness and had a strong family history of psychiatric illness (his father had committed suicide and his sister was chronically psychotic). He reluctantly sought a second opinion with a colleague who concurred with the recommendation. For a period of weeks after the consultation, Dr. R put forth evidence of his new found health, certain that the knowledge he had gained when depressed would insulate him from further illness. He could only fleetingly entertain the idea that the very fact that he continued to visit the therapist suggested he might not feel so certain of his prognosis. The treatment ended when the patient expressed the belief that his illnesses were a thing of the past and that preventive treatment would interfere with creativity. For this patient, the narcissistic gratification of his hypomania made prophylactic treatment a threat by virtue of its effectiveness. There was no way to cultivate a therapeutic alliance with him and the treatment came to an end.

For Dr. R, the medication became threatening only after it had alleviated a painful and life-threatening depression. His attitude about the medicine was state dependent. His inability to accept the need for prophylaxis was due to its impact on his self-esteem (prominently linked to a denial of his vulnerability and the pleasure of his creative abilities).

It is not only the narcissistic patient who will experience medication as a threat to his sense of self (Busch & Auchincloss, 1995). If the medication fosters a significant change in one's long-standing and stable way of being in the world, this will also trigger anxiety and distress. Patients with chronic anxiety and depression who gain significant relief from pharmacotherapy will often struggle to create a coherent narrative about their "better than well" change (Dumit, 2003). Often a period of mourning occurs due to the loss of one's "old" self. Patients will also struggle with whether their improvement is "real" or "artificial" because medication is involved, reflecting the tendency to falsely dichotomize, discussed in chapter 2. Our view is that medication does not, by definition, create a true or false self. It can alter an individual's sense of self and no doubt reflects a state-related change—that is, a self on medicine. Whether an individual sees this as a closer approximation to his genuine self or not is a matter of interpretation frequently colored by unconscious fantasy.

MEDICATION AS A THREAT TO THE TRANSFERENCE RELATIONSHIP

While an individual's fears of damage by medication will often fruitfully be explored within the transference, at other times the threat may be to the transference relationship itself. To protect the relationship, the use of medication must be fended off. As discussed in chapter 3, when medication is recommended during the course of a dynamic treatment, some patients will feel narcissistically injured and fear they have disappointed the therapist because verbal therapy has been insufficient.

Sometimes the avoidance of medication can take dramatic form. Roose and Gabbard (1997) present a case of a woman in analysis who repelled the analyst's recommendation that she have a trial of an antidepressant by becoming pregnant not once but twice. It was only after the acting out occurred that the meaning of her resistance to medication could be understood. She feared that if she were not flawed by her depressive state that her tie to her husband, and by association to her analyst, would be jeopardized. Refusing medication to stay depressed served to alleviate this anxiety. It was only after she felt protected from her own negative feelings toward her husband by creating a family that she was able to accept a medication trial and explore these issues. This exploration also involved addressing her fantasy that being depressed could keep her attached to the analyst, whom she feared losing.

For some patients, medication will be used in the service of threatening the transference relationship, rather than fended off in order to preserve it. Swoiskin (2001) argues that for this reason the introduction of medication can interfere with full psychic integration for some patients and that this factor should be considered when deciding whether to recommend medication. We believe that a patient's defensive use of medication is something that should be interpreted and not used as a basis to withhold medication, a point of view encouraged by Cabaniss (2001). Still, we concur with Swoiskin and others who have noted the introduction of medication can be employed for defensive purposes, typically to avoid the exploration of meaning. The patient will seize on drug therapy to conclude that his suffering resides in the realm of his biology—as opposed to his psyche. At times, it will be presented as prima facie evidence, an open-and-shut case supported by the use of medicine and its positive effect.

The clinician who anticipates this possibility will be in a better position to focus on the defensive aspects of this view. The appropriate tack is to support the patient's view that there is a biological basis for his suffering while exploring the need to hold onto this view as the sole explanation. Presumably, the clinician will have generated hypotheses based on the patient's story to support the appropriateness of an exploratory approach. An empathic exploration of the anxieties at play in embracing an additional psychological point of view will often diminish the resistance to psychotherapy.

Ms. S was a 25-year-old woman with panic disorder who, after a successful earlier period of brief psychotherapy for panic disorder, relapsed coincident with having to make a decision about whether to marry her boyfriend, whom she experienced as abusive. Aware that medication could be used for panic disorder, she requested a drug trial in conjunction with psychotherapy. Sertraline brought her substantial symptomatic relief.

Ms. S: Zoloft has worked wonders! This must mean my symptoms are biological. Like the ads on television say, I must have a chemical imbalance that the drug is helping correct. I am glad you agreed to give me the medicine.

Therapist: I'm pleased you're feeling better. I'd like to better understand how you interpret your improvement, given all the turmoil you were in before coming to see me.

Ms. S: Well, that's what I am thinking. Why am I here? It was the panic attacks that brought me to see you in the first place, and you've helped me a lot so that I am no longer having attacks.

Therapist: Yes, the medication has clearly helped you. But I think you may be frightened to consider that your symptoms were also linked to your confusion about whether to marry a man you felt was abusive.

Ms. S: (annoyed) Fortunately, I'm not feeling anxious anymore.

Therapist: That is fortunate. However, we need to continue to explore your conflicted feelings about your relationship, in part to further reduce your vulnerability to panic and also because, however symptom-free you are from anxiety, you are clearly not content in the predicament you describe being in.

Ms. S: I'm upset with you. I think … because I would rather think that the pill is a cure-all. It would be so much easier. Talking about personal stuff is hard for me, and I'd rather not. But this has been an issue that keeps coming up, and I know I have to get a handle on this to be happy. I wish a pill would make it all okay.

The therapist validated the role of the medicine in helping Ms. S to feel better. His comments conveyed an impression that he did not see medicine and talk therapy as competing. This made it relatively easy for him to focus on the patient's defensive use of the medication to try to shut down the exploratory process. The subsequent psychotherapeutic work clarified that the patient had an intense fear of abandonment that derived from repeated experiences of abandonment by her father throughout her childhood and adolescence that culminated in his moving halfway around the world. Within the transference, her fear of being left was dealt with by a reluctance to allow herself to get deeply connected and dependent on the therapist.

MEDICATION AS TRANSITIONAL OBJECT

Transitional phenomena are frequently evident in patients who use medication. Rather than reflecting the anticipation of harm as seen with nocebo phenomena, these patients will invest the medicine with positive meaning. Hausner (1985) relates the soothing function of the transitional object to one aspect of the placebo response. He suggests that primitive idealization of the physician fuels the wish for merger and derives from the early infant–mother relationship. Separations in vulnerable individuals can be experienced as traumatic, setting the stage for medicine to be used as a transitional object.

While the yearning for a powerful healer fuels the establishment of the transitional object, its use can simultaneously defend against individuation. In extreme cases, the medicine can take the form of a fetishistic object. Greenacre (1977) spoke of a "pill fetish" as the ritualistic use of bedtime medicine paralleling the transitional object of the child. She described this phenomenon for the reassuring pill as a "pseudoaddiction." As outlined by Winnocott (1967), a degree of object constancy must develop for the transitional object to be relinquished. When the environment is highly unstable, the pill cannot be invested with the security that it otherwise provides; once it is invested, it cannot be divested of this meaning without further stabilization of the patient's inner world.

The anxious patient who struggles with separation issues and fears of loss and destruction will often make use of medication as a transitional object (TO). Adelman (1985) observes that patients with primitive character pathology will frequently experience medication in this way. The therapist, like the pill, can be invested with characteristics that emanate largely from the patient's needs and not from the therapist. We observe that TO use cuts across a wide spectrum of psychopathology and can be observed in relatively high-functioning patients with anxiety disorders to those with significant borderline pathology. Whatever its cause, the clinician can observe this function by what the patient says. Often it is the presence of a pill in a pocket or even a prescription that brings comfort to a patient.

Ms. T was a 30-year-old woman who had previously been in treatment for panic disorder and major depression that had been successfully treated with intensive psychotherapy and sertraline 2 years prior. She returned 7 months after her son was born, with recurrent panic attacks and depressive symptoms that coincided with her return to work. There was a resurgence of anxiety around separation and loss, an anxiety that derived from the sudden death of her father from a massive heart attack when she was an adolescent and away from home with her classmates on a holiday vacation. Within 2 months of returning to treatment (she was in psychotherapy and receiving sertraline and lorazepam), she was feeling markedly better. This coincided with the typical therapeutic effect of the SSRI and focused dynamic work on her panic attacks.

In particular, her growing and intensely pleasurable attachment to her child gave way to full-blown panic attacks that, when explored, were linked to the catastrophic fear of losing her son as she had unexpectedly lost her father some 20 years prior. At one point, she commented that she was feeling much better and thought it must be due to the medicine beginning to work. Exploring the wishful element of this attribution, it became clear that pills were certain; they could not die or leave her. She spoke of the lorazepam in her pocketbook and joked that anyone who tried to mug her would be in trouble. She said this while fully aware that the low dose of lorazepam she took was probably not playing a significant role in her relief. As she spoke she reached into her pocket and took out a handkerchief she always carried around that belonged to her mother. Slightly embarrassed, she took out a wet diaper she had held onto after leaving her son to come to the therapy appointment.

She then took out tissues she had taken from the therapist's office the prior session. She said she kept them with her from session to session. The therapist suggested she did this as a way of staying connected to him. She tearfully spoke of how she kept the contents of her father's wallet, a mournful reminder of his death. She also noted that when she was pregnant she was panic free; she never felt alone. Even riding an elevator, something she typically avoided doing, was easy for her when she felt the presence of the baby inside her. Separation, which brought up anxiety, frustration, and anger, was eliminated during this psychically blissful state. As she left the session, she grabbed a few tissues and wiped her eyes.

For Ms. T, lorazepam, prescribed "as needed" while the sertraline was being titrated, was being used as a transitional object. She also used tissues as well as other objects in this way to keep her connected to important figures she had lost or feared losing. Her fears of dependency and helplessness were poignantly illustrated in the way in which the fetus had helped to diminish her anxiety. Once the therapist identifies that a drug is being used as a transitional object, he can consider when and how to interpret its use. Given the fact that panic patients are typically frightened of loss in the setting of fearing their own aggression, it is often helpful for these patients to explore the TO function. More will be said about panic patients in chapter 8.

Transitional object use typically refers to something the patient is doing with the drug, not the clinician. However, sometimes the analyst will support a drug's use in this way because he needs a reprieve from the intensity of analytic work. This reflects a transference–countertransference enactment, the analysis of which can move the treatment forward in important ways.

Ms. U was a woman in her mid-30s in analysis for chronic anxiety, hypochondriasis, masochism, and fear of intimacy. She had a highly disturbed childhood with a psychotic mother who was physically and verbally abusive and a father who had abandoned the family to marry a much younger woman when the patient was 5. In the second year of the analysis, the analyst had a death in his family and cancelled his hours for 2 weeks. When he returned to work, the patient told him she had obtained a sleeping pill, actually a low dose of sinequan, from her internist to help her sleep. The analyst renewed the medication twice while analyzing the patient's need for it. The willingness of the analyst to do this in part reflected his countertransference need to fend off the patient's rage while he was grieving. She spoke of the pill as her "security blanket" and invested it with oral meaning—"pacifier," "battery juice"—helping the "negativity to bounce off." She felt it kept her from "drowning." She offered to "support" the analyst if someone had died and recalled all the times she tried to keep her mother going by being happy.

As the analyst moved through his grief he regained his interpretive function, first focusing on the maternal element (that she felt that, just as she could not depend upon her mother, she could not depend upon the analyst) and then on the paternal (feeling abandoned by the analyst as she had been by her father). After the first interpretation, she dreamed of going on a murder rampage after being disappointed by a man. After the second interpretation, she associated to a memory of almost drowning by walking on thin ice behind her father's house, enraged at him and feeling rejected. The idea the medicine would keep her from drowning was associatively linked to this memory. She subsequently developed severe hand pain on Father's Day and soaked her hands in ice. The analyst interpreted the pain as a somatic expression of rage she feared verbalizing. Coincident with her increased sense of safety with her aggression in the transference, she was able to discontinue the use of sinequan after 2½ months.

In this vignette, the analysand first instituted the use of the transitional object when the analyst precipitously interrupted the treatment. Then the analyst encouraged and perpetuated its use while his capacity to be available was limited by his grief. The sinequan gave both patient and analyst something to hold onto. The patient's ability to let go of its use coincided with the analyst's presence being rediscovered through his ability to interpret the patient's terror of her hostility within the transference.

Not all psychological dependency on medication need have transitional features. The positive meanings invested in medication are also sustained by culture and history. The soothing function of the drug may pertain to the curative potency of doctors, medicine, and science. Some patients may overvalue the pill because it is associated with a connection to "real" doctoring, so the medication reassures them that the analyst is a "real" doctor who does know what is wrong with them and can prescribe something that, talking aside, will help them feel better.

MEDICATION AS OBJECT

Psychotic patients, displaying concrete thinking, can imbue medication with meaning that reflects primary process thought. For example,

Gutheil (1982) has described patients expressing preferences based on the projected gender of the drug ("Mo" [short for Moban] being a male drug; "Stella" [short for Stelazine] being a female drug). Tutter (2006) elaborates on how the personification of a drug can occur among high-functioning patients. She points out that medication is ideally suited to take on the characteristics of an object. It is given by the object of the analyst (or in split treatment by the pharmacotherapist) and can be invested with intentionality and personhood.

The personification of the medicine can reflect an extension of the predominant transference to the analyst or, by the use of splitting, a defense against the awareness of a transference trend. For example, a pill can symbolize poison or the poisonous mother. The experience of the pill as poison, while depersonalized, makes more apparent that it is the prescriber who, by association, is the poisoning mother. The defensive personification of the medicine may create a safe space that permits analysis of frightening transference fantasies. Such reactions can occur when the medicine is invested with affectionate (or libidinal) meaning as well. Tutter (2006) also observes that transferences to the medicine can change during the course of treatment. For example, the medication may represent the patient, the therapist, or significant figures from the patient's past; the meaning of medication is not static. Her report of one such patient will be discussed in chapter 6.

It is unclear whether the relative paucity of reports in the literature on medication as an object reflects a countertransference blind spot to its presence. An alternative viewpoint is that an analyst who employs a more object-relational perspective is more likely to evoke this kind of meaning than one who works differently.

SHIFTING ATTITUDES TOWARD MEDICATION FROM WORKING THROUGH CHANGE

As observed before, the meaning of medication is not static. In addition to the possibility of medication taking on different object representations, patients' attitudes toward medication can shift during critical moments in therapy. When change is frightening, this can result in increased defensive activity with medication employed as a vehicle to express that defensiveness. Alternatively, shifting attitudes can express a consolidation of significant emotional growth. The following vignettes are illustrative.

Mr. V had been engaged in an intensive psychotherapy three times per week while receiving buproprion for dysthymia, a regimen that had been stable from the start. He presented with an entrenched belief that relationships with women would always end badly for him and linked this to an experience with a mentally ill mother who alternated between emotionally suffocating and abandoning the patient. Productive therapeutic work revealed the degree to which he had blamed himself for his mother's shortcomings while repeatedly engaging women in ways that guaranteed the demise of the relationship after some period of time. As the defensive aspect of this behavior was elaborated (he would end involvements before feeling smothered or left), the idea that he had created a risk-free life shifted to a view that he risked depriving himself of the possibility of romantic love.

The patient subsequently dated a woman whom he perceived as narcissistically preoccupied, suggesting the use of a vibrator as he was going to penetrate her. The patient lost his erection, became mortified, and subsequently expressed the worry that this problem, of new onset, would now permeate future involvements. He felt somewhat relieved after analysis revealed a pattern of self-blame and a defensive turning of anger against himself. He subsequently was able to identify several aspects of the woman's behavior that suggested she was self-centered. Some weeks later he began dating again and expressed apprehension around sexual functioning. He noted only in passing that he was taking a drug for alopecia known to have an impact on libido. The therapist raised for consideration that, given the possible overdetermined nature of his sexual symptom, he chose to continue to take a drug that would serve to reinforce an anxiety he purportedly wanted to be rid of.

In the past, he had come to see the various ways he made "pre-emptive strikes" against women, planning his exit upon first meeting them. After considering his apparent lack of motivation to stop a drug that could be contributing to the problem, he wondered if, once again, albeit in a different way, he was expressing his anxiety around intimacy. The symptom expressed a downward displacement, onto his genitals, of a fear of being inadequate with a woman. By not doing what he could to diminish the risk from a drug (used to deal with a fear of inadequacy due to hair loss), he could justify exiting the relationship by not entering it! The patient decided to stop the medication at this point.

For Mr. V there was heightened defensiveness evident in wanting to stay on a drug that could be creating sexual problems at a time when he was more in touch with the desire for closeness. For Ms. W, described next, her shifting attitude toward medicine was a palpable sign of an important growth within the therapeutic relationship.

Ms. W was a middle-aged teacher with a long history of schizoaffective illness characterized by severe bouts of depression (requiring ECT) and paranoia. Her medication included escitalopram, lamotrigine, and olanzapine. When euthymic, she struggled with profound feelings of self-hatred and emptiness that were linked to severe physical abuse by her mother. She entered a combined treatment and over many years of intensive psychotherapy, together with complex medication regimens, began to feel more alive and less terrified of the world.

This dynamic shift was forged largely through work in the transference. Her fear of being hateful and destructive like her mother alternated with powerful paranoid trends, where the therapist was the terrifying and sadistic mother who would not tolerate her complaints or autonomy. Feeling like an "empty shell" protected her from the terror of being hatefully attacked or attacking. She tended to be passive and compliant with authority figures.

She often complained of feeling tired but seemed to work tirelessly. Her professional life was all encompassing, though in the last year she had begun to pursue other interests like going to the museum and reading for leisure. Seemingly out of the blue, Ms. W came in one day and requested a trial of modafinil (Provigil) to help with daytime sleepiness and fatigue. She had recalled that, one year prior, the therapist had discussed this option but quickly dismissed it because it was a relatively new agent for psychiatric patients. He had also thought to himself that her effort to be more alert was driven by a masochistic wish to work compulsively and did not derive from a significant side effect, though he knew there was no definitive way of parsing this out.

The request itself represented a significant and highly uncharacteristic step for Ms. W. While she fleetingly became frightened that she had aggressively transgressed a boundary ("if you thought it would be helpful, clearly you would have already given it to me"), she understood that she had come to feel safe enough to be assertive with the therapist. She could reveal what was on her mind, not to attack or provoke, but to facilitate his helping her to feel better. Medication became a vehicle for this transference shift.

The therapist subsequently considered why he had withheld modafinil from the patient. He had downplayed in his mind that work was an important source of gratification for her and had made a clinical judgment not to engage in a sadomasochistic enactment (helping her gain energy to work more hours). It was only after she had received a trial of modafinil that he realized he had inadvertently engaged in the enactment he was seeking to avoid by having withheld the medication. She had a robust response to the drug and noted a significant increase in her energy level and increased clarity of thought that served to make her more efficient, not masochistically more entrenched in working.

It is probable that the clinician was blinded to a side effect he had caused his patient because it appeared masked by significant masochistic pathology, the attenuation of which freed the patient and therapist to manage the side effect more effectively, while establishing an important shift in the transference. Independent of the positive effect of the drug, the request crystallized out years of work in the transference where an insistent need to view the therapist as a terrifying, sadistic authority made genuine contact and mutuality difficult. There are very few times when a patient has the opportunity to make an explicit request of the analyst to be given something. Medication is one of them. Her request signaled a turning point in the clinical work.

MEDICATION AS A COUNTERTRANSFERENCE ENACTMENT

There are times when medication is meaningful because its use signifies the presence of countertransference. Subtle manifestations of this include the case of Ms. U, where she and the analyst used the pill as a kind of transitional object. At other times, the therapist may feel the need to fend off intense affect within the transference. Symptoms can be misdiagnosed as a primary mood disturbance, especially if the patient is frightened and evokes a similar feeling in the clinician. A common scenario is grief, where emotional pain can feel overwhelming and the clinician is vulnerable to being overcome by a sense of helplessness. Rather than functioning to contain such feelings for the patient, there is the risk that these emotions will be deemed pathological and be medicated. Important moments of change can be characterized by intense emotional pain. At the same time, the clinician has to be alert to indications of pathological mourning and potential legitimate indications for the use of antidepressants in this population.

Sometimes a therapist, in an effort to manage the medication competently, inadvertently becomes engaged in a countertransference enactment. The following vignette is illustrative. (This will be discussed in more detail in chapter 6.)

Mr. X complained of a loss of libido in the third year of his analysis, the duration of which he had been medicated with sertraline for chronic major depression. Prior to the complaint, the analyst was struck by the paucity of material related to his marriage. Because diminished libido is a known side effect of the drug, the analyst responded to the patient's request by adding buproprion, which had been reported to be helpful for some patients. He surmised that doing so might increase Mr. X's sexual desire and facilitate the analysis of this previously withheld part of his emotional life—a foreclosure the analyst regarded as, at least in part, a result of the medication.

A couple of months after buproprion was added and shortly before the analyst's August vacation, the patient became sexually involved with a woman the patient saw as young enough to be his daughter. This acting out reversed an important and traumatic aspect of his childhood. When the patient was a teenager, his mother married a man half her age who was young enough to be Mr. X's brother. The father subsequently moved far away. The analyst was both the absent father (his upcoming vacation) and an inadvertent coconspirator to the patient's acting out.

In this vignette, the analyst's effort to relieve a presumed drug side effect revealed an underlying motivation to act out in the transference. One cannot predict what would have happened if the analyst had been more alert to this possibility before prescribing. However, upon reflection, the preferred response to Mr. X's complaint would have been to explore why this particular problem was coming up at that time and not to prescribe an antidote immediately.

IS IT ALWAYS USEFUL TO EXPLORE MEANING?

The therapist can avoid a psychological exploration of matters relating to medicine or too aggressively seek it out. Awad (2001) describes two analytic patients who were treated with medication after being sent for consultation. In each case the analyst, after discussing the consultant's recommendations with the analysand, assumed the role of the prescriber. Each patient had initial reactions to the introduction of medication, and the early phase of their use was occasioned by an exploration of various transferences to the drug. However, to his surprise, Awad found that, after this initial period, issues related to the psychological meaning of the medicine did not appear either directly or, as best he could tell, in derivative form.

While it is often, even usually, helpful to the patient to explore the meaning of the medicine, there are also some patients for whom the acceptance of medication seamlessly folds into the *unobjectionable transference*. Sometimes, after a relatively brief period of analysis around the recommendation and introduction of a drug, the medication ceases to be a significant issue in the treatment. We encourage an attitude of receptive curiosity and openness around the exploration of meaning. The clinician benefits from being neither overly aggressive about nor phobically avoidant of exploring meaning. We argue for the ongoing relevance of the exploration of meaning of medication for most, not all, patients receiving medication.

CONCLUDING COMMENTS

In this chapter, we have illustrated how the use of medication for patients in psychotherapy and psychoanalysis can provide unique opportunities for dynamic exploration. The clinician who manages his negative countertransference about drug use will be in a good position to see a patient's need for medicine as an opportunity to further the psychotherapeutic process. This deepening derives not only from relieving symptoms that can make introspective work difficult but also from the various meanings patients attach to medicine. Cultural factors will inevitably come into play and be recruited by patients to serve their defensive needs. The placebo effect will be explored based on the depth of treatment, while the anticipation of threat (nocebo effect) will often require investigation, especially through work in the transference.

Transitional phenomena are common in anxious patients and those with primitive pathology and can create opportunities for deepening analysis and encouraging a process of internalization. Medication can take on various object representations that change over time due to an evolving therapeutic process. In some cases, medicine is meaningful because its use either moves the process ahead by relieving an obstruction or impedes it by serving resistance. Important transference and countertransference enactments can emerge around medication issues.

5

Clinical Values of Combined Treatment

The ways in which medication can make psychotherapy more productive and in which psychotherapy can help patients accept the need for medication will be described in this chapter. Patients with significant anxious or depressive symptoms will often benefit from or need medication to work effectively in psychotherapy because their difficulties with concentration and motivation can disrupt their ability to utilize the therapist's comments (Wright & Hollifield, 2006). In addition, patients presenting with personality disorders, such as narcissistic and borderline disorder, who appear to be resistant to psychotherapeutic intervention can have underlying affective or cognitive disorders that exacerbate their symptomatology (Oldham, 2006); relief of affective instability and low self-esteem with medication, for example, can sometimes aid these patients in tolerating exploration of conflict and painful feelings.

Psychotherapy can help in addressing resistances to medication in cases in which it is indicated, but patients are unwilling to take it or do not take it consistently (Book, 1987). This can be accomplished particularly by exploring the meanings of medications to the patient (Busch & Auchincloss, 1995), as discussed in chapter 4. Feelings of shame about needing medication, fears of not being in control, resistances to "authority," and a variety of other conflicts that can disrupt compliance and interfere with treatment can be usefully brought to light and addressed in a way that eases patients' fears.

MEDICATION AS AN AID TO PSYCHOTHERAPY

Treatment of Affective and Cognitive Symptoms That Disrupt Psychotherapy

Medication for Affective Disorders In many instances, patients can suffer depressive, anxious, or psychotic symptoms that significantly disrupt their ability to participate in psychotherapy (depressive and anxiety disorders will be addressed in more depth in chapter 8). In addition to the negative impact of problems with motivation and concentration, these patients will tend to accept catastrophic fantasies as representing reality or will be able to reality test them only intermittently. These preoccupations disrupt the patient's capacity to employ an observing ego and ally with the therapist in exploring the psychological origins of his symptoms. For instance, if a depressed patient is convinced that his situation is hopeless, he would see little value in exploring the hopelessness as a fantasy. Medication can reduce the intensity of these ideas, limiting the threat the patient experiences or reducing the frequency of a preoccupation. The inability to ease a persistent and catastrophic preoccupation through psychotherapy is an indication to consider medication and to evaluate the patient for the presence of other symptoms of an affective or psychotic disorder.

For instance, Ms. Y, a 38-year-old woman, presented with feelings of worthlessness associated with vegetative symptoms of depression. Because of her low self-esteem, Ms. Y allowed herself to be mistreated by men in her life, including her father, her boss, and her boyfriend. For instance, her boss would criticize her for her not doing her job as an administrative secretary fast enough and make comments suggesting she was incapable and inept, in spite of giving her positive yearly evaluations and salary increases. Ms. Y accepted this treatment because she felt she was "stupid" and unattractive and therefore deserved these attacks. She occasionally felt angry and wanted to confront her boss with the injustice of his comments, but this feeling was infrequent. In addition, she feared addressing these problems because she was concerned that it would lead him to attack and humiliate her further.

Ms. Y was begun on medication, but it took her almost 3 months to respond to increasing doses of venlafaxine and bupropion. During this time it was difficult for Ms. Y to make progress in psychotherapy because of her recurring preoccupation with feelings of worthlessness; she took this self-assessment as a given, rather than as something to be understood. Exploring Ms. Y's background revealed that her relationship with her father mirrored that with her boss. She felt ignored and disregarded by him because he was focused on his work as a successful salesman. He tended to treat the patient, her mother, and her siblings with disdain and would have frequent temper tantrums in which he would refer to his children as "stupid" or "bumbling." Attempts to interpret the sources of her problems in relation to her father had little impact because she would say, "Well, I think he was probably right, given how I can't manage things."

When Ms. Y's depression lifted she was able to make more effective use of the therapist's observations. She no longer accepted at face value the negative comments from her boss and boyfriend, and confronting them regarding their attitude was more effective than she thought. In addition to exploring in more depth the origins of her problems in the family structure, Ms. Y revealed a period in her adolescence when she became her father's favorite and was taken with him to meet clients. Ms. Y had not presented this history when depressed, assuming it was irrelevant. Guilt that emerged from the patient's oedipal and sibling rivalry victories was profound, and Ms. Y felt a need to attack or undercut her success as a punishment. Working through this dynamic helped to free her further from self-recriminations and feelings of worthlessness.

Medication Intervention for Personality Disorders Medication intervention can relieve cognitive and affective disturbances in some patients with severe personality disorders, allowing for a more effective psychotherapeutic intervention (Oldham, 2006). As noted in chapter 1, boundaries between Axis I and Axis II disorders have become more blurred, and symptoms of what have been considered character problems have been found to overlap with affective disorders. For borderline personality disorder, recommendations have been made that medication target three symptom clusters, based on randomized controlled clinical trials: affective dysregulation (SSRIs or related antidepressants), impulsive-behavioral dyscontrol (SSRIs), and cognitive-perceptual symptoms (low-dose antipsychotic medications) (American Psychiatric Association, 2001).

Although not systematically studied, case reports suggest medication may be of value in other personality disorders (Oldham, 2006). When psychotherapists are treating patients with personality disorders, they should consider medication if symptoms appear to be disrupting therapeutic progress, or if there is comorbidity with Axis I disorders that have been found to be medication responsive. In Wylie and Wylie's (1995) metaphor (chapter 2), such symptoms may represent an obstruction from chemical factors rather than a psychologically based resistance.

Borderline Personality Disorder Vignette

Ms. Z, a 48-year-old divorced lawyer, reported a long history of recurrent major depression and symptoms consistent with borderline personality disorder. These symptoms included intense and unstable relationships alternating between extremes of idealization and devaluation, and affective instability, fluctuating among irritability, anxiety, and depression. While typically lasting only a few days, on occasion the depressive symptoms continued for more extended periods. Additionally, she demonstrated inappropriate or intense bouts of anger and temper outbursts, frantic efforts to avoid abandonment, and persistent identity disturbances surrounding career goals and types of friends desired. Various antidepressants, alone and in combination, had provided little relief for these symptoms.

Although tensions occurred with her boyfriend, Ms. Z's central source of conflict occurred with her family. Despite recurrent pledges to distance herself from her family and make efforts to "do things for [her]self," Ms. Z was repeatedly drawn back to them. She alternated between a view of her mother as exploitative, desperately needy, and overly demanding and a sense of her as legitimately asking for support, victimized by her alcoholic father's harsh criticisms and neglect. When the therapist attempted to confront Ms. Z about her alternating views, she would become enraged and devaluing of the therapist. For instance, when Ms. Z described the necessity of visiting her mother because of her mother's plight, the therapist reminded her that, typically, when she went on these visits, she left feeling outraged and exploited, her efforts to pursue her legal career and friendships thwarted. After this comment, Ms. Z became furious at the therapist for not understanding her mother's situation and the necessity of her being involved. The therapist also experienced little collaboration in his attempt to look at potential abandonment fears that drew Ms. Z back to her involvement with her family.

Ms. Z described her background as one in which she was pushed to be the mother's parent rather than her mother parenting her. If she did not respond to her mother's requests for help, her mother would become angry with her. Her mother was generally irritable, withdrawn, isolated, and frustrated with her husband. Rather than acknowledging her parental shortcomings, her mother presented herself as a victim of her husband's hurtful behavior. Her mother would either scoff at or not pursue suggestions on altering her life, such as finding her own friends and hobbies or reducing her drinking, seeming to prefer to see herself as victimized. She never left her husband, despite recurrent threats to do so. Ms. Z resented the need to be a parent rather than be taken care of, but at the same time, caretaking behaviors led her to feel an unusual sense of importance and provided a safeguard for her attachment to her mother.

After a period of more prolonged depression, agitation, and irritability, the therapist added an atypical antipsychotic, quetiapine, for relief of these symptoms and mood stabilization. Notably, the patient had not only additional relief of depression, but also reduced irritability and mood swings. This provided therapist and patient an opportunity for Ms. Z to consider her contradictory attitudes and emotional shifts with less anger at the therapist because they were less intense. Ms. Z was able to acknowledge her tendency to alternate her attitudes. She more frequently allied with the therapist in how to manage her guilty pull toward involvement with her mother. This observing ego was critical to psychotherapeutic progress.

Ms. Z: I really feel like I must visit my mother this weekend. She's miserable and my father treats her like crap. There's nothing for her to do.

Therapist: Well I think we should talk about what your feelings are and how to handle it because we know you often get upset after you go. You end up feeling drained and often depressed.

Ms. Z: That's true, but that's because my father attacks me.

Therapist: Yes, but you often feel drained and depressed about your mother. You feel somehow you're supposed to rescue her.

Ms. Z: I know what you're saying. I feel guilty if I don't go and frustrated when I do. But my mother does feel better during the time I'm there.

Therapist: I think we need to understand more about your guilt driving you. You act as though you are your mother's only option, and yet you know you have made many efforts to get her to pursue other activities.

Ms. Z: Yes. I forgot about that.

This vignette shows Ms. Z's growing capacity to integrate her various conflicts and have the capability to step back and consider them. Although the development of the observing ego is an important aspect of psychodynamic psychotherapy, Ms. Z, like other patients with symptoms of borderline personality disorder, was unable to do this until she was treated with a mood stabilizer. This ego weakness or deficit appears to have been caused at least in part by difficulty modulating her mood. Thus, medication allowed a stalemate associated with her personality disorder to be eased. Problems and struggles of the sort that preceded the mood stabilizer treatment still occurred but not nearly to the extent they did prior to the medication addition.

Narcissistic Personality Disorder Vignette

Mr. AA, a 52-year-old financial manager, presented with typical symptoms of narcissistic personality disorder, including an incessant need for admiration and rages at those he experienced as rejecting or interfering with his successes. The office where he worked suggested that he come in for evaluation because of increasing conflicts he was having with coworkers. Mr. AA was also frustrated by limitations of business rules that he felt should not apply to him. He was constantly running into conflicts with regulators at his company who felt his efforts were on the border of being illegal or unethical. Despite his awareness that his anger might get out of hand, he had little empathy for those whom he attacked, feeling they deserved it for their lax attitudes or rigid positions. Also of note, Mr. AA described a period of symptoms consistent with a major depressive episode following the death of his father 3 years previously that was treated with psychotherapy but not medication. It was following recovery from this episode, accompanied by a period of increased success, that his conflicts at work intensified.

In treatment, Mr. AA recognized that he had a problem with "overreacting," although he appeared to minimize the degree of his temper relative to what was described by coworkers at his office. However, when the therapist attempted to explore these reactions with him, he focused on justifications for his behavior, referring to subordinates who did not work efficiently, bosses who did not understand what he was doing and interfered in unnecessary ways, and errors committed by his wife that were very frustrating to him, preventing some of the few opportunities he had to relax. This externalization of his problems affected his interest in pursuing the intrapsychic origins of these reactions because he did not see his psychology as a contributing factor.

Mr. AA: I lost my temper with one of my assistants yesterday.

Therapist: What happened?

Mr. AA: Well, deals need to get done very quickly in my office. That's how we get our business and stay ahead of the pack. When someone decides he's going to leave early and not complete the job, it puts us all in a bad position.

Therapist: Yes. Well, I can understand your being upset, but at least when we've talked about it in the past, losing your temper means screaming and insulting someone.

Mr. AA: Yes. I know everyone's on my case about that, but if it's necessary to put some fear into these people and get them to do the work, I'll yell at them.

Given the degree of the problem he was struggling with, Mr. AA raised the question of whether antidepressants might be helpful. Although there were not definitive indications of an Axis I disorder, Mr. AA had persistent insomnia, and periodic anxious preoccupations (from incidents when he felt frustrated or disparaged at work), in addition to irritability, along with the prior history of major depression. A sertraline trial was initiated, and Mr. AA reported a reduction in his irritability, insomnia, and anxious preoccupation.

With the relief of the intensity of Mr. AA's anger, the therapist could more easily engage him in looking at psychological sources of his irritability and anxiety. Mr. AA considered the idea that he was reacting to insecurity and low self-esteem in his constant feelings that others did not adequately recognize his talents or respond to his demands. Therapist and patient began to explore his background for sources of these problems. Mr. AA described an early life experience of being socially, academically, and athletically successful. However, he became distressed by increasing conflict between his parents in his early adolescence, with his mother expressing frustration about being a homemaker and wanting to pursue a career and his father demanding that she stay at home and take care of the children. When he was 15 his parents split up. Mr. AA felt angry and depressed, and he began to draw back from his studies and become more rebellious with authority figures.

His problems intensified when his mother spent increasing time pursuing a career and his father quickly remarried. His father's new wife had two small children, and his father expected that he readily accept his new family and refer to his stepmother as "mom." Mr. AA felt like a second-class citizen and reacted angrily to his father's pressures, leading to a rift between them. Although he was able to reengage in his studies, Mr. AA's feelings of neglect and anger persisted.

After reviewing these details, Mr. AA was able to consider a connection between his adolescent disappointments and his frustration with bosses, subordinates, and his wife, including his feelings that he was unrecognized and not adequately responded to.

Mr. AA: My secretary brought up that I had been nasty to her and I realized it was true. It wasn't anything like I had done before, but I apologized to her.

Therapist: What do you think happened?

Mr. AA: Well, I was feeling a lot of pressure on this deal, and I guess I began to worry that it would fall through. I started to feel that I might be in trouble with the firm.

Therapist: We have been discussing how you fear being excluded by your partners as you felt excluded by your father. Do you think this was playing a role?

Mr. AA: Yes. That's why I mentioned it. I recognize more of what you're saying. I was aware that I was worried they would attack me, and I guess I took it out on her.

In this instance, as in others, the reduction in the intensity of Mr. AA's rage allowed him to consider the underlying insecurity that triggered it. In this sense, as with Ms. Z, symptoms that could be seen as part of Mr. AA's personality disorder were relieved with the medication. Although Mr. AA may well have eventually engaged in this exploration with therapy alone, it appeared that medication and the decrement in his anger sped up this process. It is also possible that, if not given medication, Mr. AA could have dropped out of treatment, frustrated that the therapist did not understand the problems that others were causing and feeling blamed by the therapist's efforts to pursue intrapsychic sources of his symptoms.

Reaction to Medication as a Basis for Psychotherapeutic Exploration

Medication treatment raises issues that may be addressed in psychotherapy that can otherwise be difficult to access. Clinicians should be alert to these opportunities, rather than segregating responses to medication to a nonpsychotherapeutic realm. The following vignette demonstrates how exploration of a side effect allowed the clinician to address the transference in a patient usually resistant to such efforts.

Mr. BB was a 45-year-old businessman with a history of chronic severe depression. Along with his symptoms, he had long-standing difficulties with keeping track of his finances and furnishing his home. He was highly demanding of himself and others, and his criticisms limited his ability to maintain close relationships. He experienced authority as rigid, harsh, and arbitrary and would respond with a passive–aggressive stance that tended to trigger attacks by others he viewed as authorities. Notable in Mr. BB's history was his relationship with his father, whom he experienced as demeaning and critical, often referring to the patient as stupid or incapable. His mother was emotionally disconnected and of little help in dealing with his father. His father was a prominent businessman who was a philanthropist, and his mother and those in the community tended to view him as a "hero." Mr. BB had difficulty integrating this hero status with his father's harshness.

In addition, over the years the father had become involved in shady business dealings that eventually led to legal investigations. His father became increasingly involved in substance use and collapsed and died in front of Mr. BB when he was 13. Mr. BB primarily felt relieved by this, but at a deeper level felt terribly guilty, with a notion that he had "killed" his father. Over the course of psychotherapy, Mr. BB came to understand that these events and his attitude toward his father evolved into his views of authority as well as his passive–aggressive struggle, along with his inability to feel safe about "growing up" by being effective in his finances and the care of his home.

Despite ongoing progress in addressing these issues in psychotherapy, Mr. BB had difficulty acknowledging transference feelings. The therapist attempted to address this resistance to the transference in relation to the threat that Mr. BB felt voicing feelings that he feared would cause the therapist to attack, reject or ignore him and concerns that he would damage the therapist. Mr. BB was able to accept these issues intellectually, but still had trouble identifying these fantasies. A breakthrough came in exploring the patient's failure to obtain a lithium level over a 3-month period, in spite of the therapist's directive to do so.

Therapist: I think at this point we need to look at why you haven't obtained a lithium level. It's obvious that some kind of struggle is going on.

Mr. BB: Well. I guess you're right at this point. I mean I could say before that I was too busy, but I really have had time lately.

Therapist: I wonder how you feel about this occurring with me, particularly since you often deny having feelings about our relationship.

However, this is the same kind of delaying and passive behavior we've often noted occurring with others.

Mr. BB: Well, I do think I'm irritated because the lithium hasn't really done that much for me. I don't know if I want to bother checking it. But I know I'm also worried you're going to get furious with me for not checking it, just like my father would start attacking me.

Therapist: I certainly think your ideas make sense, and I agree the lithium has not done much so far. Of course, this is why we want to check the level. But I think we need to understand more about why you are behaving in ways that may trigger the attack that you fear.

Mr. BB: Well. I guess I wonder whether you really want me to do well. My father indicated he wanted me to be academically successful. But he was always intent on proving that I was stupid.

Therapist: So, you feel that I'll attack you whether you get the lithium level or not.

Mr. BB: Yes. I guess so.

In this instance Mr. BB could no longer ignore that he was behaving in ways that were similar to how he behaved with others. He was able to look at his passive expression of anger at the therapist and his fear that the therapist would attack him for his poor compliance. Additionally, Mr. BB learned that he worried that the therapist would criticize him if he took proper care of himself by obtaining the level. Subsequently, Mr. BB acknowledged that he preferred to engage the therapist as a punitive "father" because it was better than feeling alone or cut off, as he felt with his mother. This breakthrough surrounding medication helped create an atmosphere for ongoing transference interpretation.

PSYCHOTHERAPY AS AN AID TO TAKING MEDICATION

Patients often struggle with taking medication, related to negative emotional reactions to medication, discomfort with side effects, reactions to the doctor prescribing them, and the meanings of medication for them. Such reactions can trigger noncompliance, considered to be a common problem in medication treatment (Riba & Tasman, 2006). By elucidating these reactions, psychotherapy can often temper interfering factors, increasing the likelihood of an effective psychopharmacological intervention.

Psychotherapy as an Aid to Tolerating Side Effects

Side effects are a common factor affecting patients' compliance with medication and add to negative transference reactions to the treating doctor or psychotherapist. However, patients vary greatly in their tolerance of side effects (see the nocebo discussion in chapter 4), and the meaning of medication and experience of it in the transference may greatly affect patients' levels of discomfort. Exploring and understanding these psychological factors may help in tolerance of side effects.

For instance, Ms. CC's depressive symptoms, accompanied by some paranoia, responded well to treatment with sertraline, up to 200 mg/day and haloperidol 2 mg/day. Attempts to taper either medication were ineffective. Ms. CC reported that although the medication had been enormously helpful to her, she noticed that she no longer had periods in which she felt enthusiastic, creative, and almost overly positive about her talents and capabilities. Although this suggested the presence of a bipolar variant, she did not describe any accompanying hypomanic or manic symptoms during the periods in which she felt this way.

She missed these excited feelings, especially since most of the time she felt inhibited about pursuing the writing career she desired and angry about having to look for a job she felt was beneath her capabilities in order to support herself. As she tended not to get these jobs, often by not pursuing them aggressively, she was forced to ask her father for support, something she found to be humiliating.

However, further investigation revealed that she was quite conflicted about these issues. She felt that throughout her life her father had undermined her efforts to be successful by criticizing or demeaning her. He stated that she was not smart enough to be a writer and would make some man "a good wife," a goal greatly at odds with her feminist views. She reported that this attitude had gone back many years, including her father's negative comments about her intelligence in grade school. In addition, she felt that her father did not financially or emotionally support her subsequent efforts to go to graduate school. In contrast, her mother would get "whatever she needed" for clothes and for her own hobbies despite not working. Thus, Ms. CC was angry about needing to pursue a job and passive aggressively took a long time to obtain one, achieving some satisfaction in getting back at her father by forcing him to pay for her living expenses.

As Ms. CC complained about her presumed side effect, her therapist stated that he understood she was troubled about this symptom, but was curious about what might be helpful in addressing her concerns, especially given the benefit of the medication. On exploration, it emerged that Ms. CC was experiencing the medication and the therapist as undermining her, just as her father did, by disallowing access to her flights of fancy that she claimed helped her to write.

Ms. CC: The medication definitely helps, but I'm really frustrated that I'm missing my creative experiences.

Therapist: It's like what I'm giving you both helps and undermines you.

Ms. CC: Yes. I didn't want to blame you, but when I think about it, I realize I am angry with you.

Therapist: It does sound like I'm representing your father, particularly as you see me as interrupting your creativity.

Ms. CC: That's true. As I've said, my father was very much against my writing career.

Therapist: Well, I think we can continue to look for medication adjustments that will help you, but I think there are other issues that are blocking your creativity as well.

Following this exchange, Ms. CC's distress at this side effect diminished, and the pursuit of other conflicts surrounding her writing helped her to steadily become more productive.

Compliance Affected by Struggles With Authority

Although authority struggles will often occur as part of a psychotherapy and benefit from exploration, medication treatment may be more likely to precipitate these issues. Authority conflicts can be triggered by the more directive or authoritative stance taken by the psychoanalyst in recommending or monitoring medication (see chapter 3). In reaction to this stance, patients can make efforts to compete with or undermine the prescribing physician's authority. This can be enacted by discontinuation of medication, self-medication via dosage reduction or increase, or directly challenging the therapist's recommendations about medication.

For instance, Mr. DD routinely pushed doses higher than the doctor's recommendation. This reflected not only his frustration with the limited impact of medication on his symptoms but also a struggle for control and a wish to undermine the therapist. Mr. DD wanted to be able to say that his changes in medication doses were more effective and achieved results faster than what the therapist was suggesting. Often, however, Mr. DD would end up struggling with more side effects or, in one instance, a toxic reaction to a higher dose.

Mr. DD described an early period of his life when he was very close to his father, who was affectionate and responsive. He experienced his mother as cold and disinterested. In addition, his father demeaned her, referring to her as incompetent. As his adolescence approached, the behavior of his father changed: He became more distant and critical of the patient. In particular, he wanted him to participate in "manly" activities, such as football, which the patient did not enjoy and was not interested in. Mr. DD felt hurt and angered by his father's behavior. Rather than athletics, the patient wanted to play the flute in the school band. Although Mr. DD did not recall if he picked this activity as a way to rebel against his father, they entered into an increasing struggle over it. His father refused to buy his son an adequate quality of flute needed to be in the band and would not pay for lessons. Mr. DD held his ground by making little effort in football, eventually being cut from the team. Their relationship grew increasingly distant, and Mr. DD described little sadness upon his father's death when the patient was 17.

Mr. DD's struggles with authority became a pattern in his life. At jobs he would become frustrated at the demanding behavior of his bosses. He would then become passive–aggressive, stonewalling on projects, and disparage the boss to others. Eventually, Mr. DD would be fired, following which he would experience a severe episode of depression. Despite his acknowledgment of this pattern, he could not seem to stop getting into conflicts on the job. He entered therapy, but his therapist wanted to refer him out due to the complexity of his psychopharmacology and for occasional noncompliance. The therapist also reported a sense that Mr. DD was more interested in fighting than in looking to improve.

When Mr. DD entered treatment with a new psychiatrist, he was prepared for a struggle because he felt hurt and angry about the termination of treatment by his prior therapist, which was readily linked to his rejection by his father. Mr. DD seemed determined to fight with his new psychiatrist's recommendations about therapy and medications. He debated the value of combined treatment, about which he had done some reading, and whether psychodynamic psychotherapy was appropriate for him. Additionally, he made medication changes without telling his therapist, as described earlier. The therapist pointed out to Mr. DD that it seemed more important for him to struggle than make progress in his treatment.

Therapist: It feels like you are more interested in debating medication with me than in taking it according to the prescription.

Mr. DD: Well, the way you prescribe the medication it takes forever for me to get on it. I'm just trying to speed things up. I don't think you get that I'm having a lot of difficulty with depression.

Therapist: I think we need to talk more about your sense that I don't get your problems or that I'm not competent to treat them, as it sounds like your experiences with your mother. However, there has been more than one time when you've pushed the dose too quickly and its created problems for you.

Mr. DD: Well, you have a point there about incompetence. That does remind me of my mother. I hope you're more capable than that. And yet, I don't seem to be getting better.

Therapist: I think we need to explore this further. It sounds very frightening to put yourself under the care of someone else.

Fear of an authority's incompetence emerged as an important dynamic, not only in Mr. DD's conflict about medication but also with his occupational conflicts. Mr. DD felt that he could not trust an authority to manage a situation properly and needed to take over the job himself. As exploration proceeded, the therapist identified several additional sources of Mr. DD's rebellious behavior. One aspect was his fear that his autonomy would be undermined, with a need to assert himself to avoid submission. Another component was an effort to engage the therapist in a struggle rather than experience rejection or the absence of a relationship. Mr. DD also wanted to win in a competition and defeat the therapist as a rival. He revealed that he had wanted to be a psychiatrist, but his grades were not adequate for medical school. Exploring these factors helped Mr. DD feel safer about following medication prescriptions.

Compliance Issues Related to Shame

Patients can experience feelings of shame related to their need for medication. These feelings can be associated with attitudes toward being ill, including having a mental illness. As noted in chapter 4, cultural factors may play a role in such experiences. Additionally, shame can be triggered by a sense of being "out of control" with regard to feelings and behaviors and requiring medication to attain control, or fearing medication will cause a loss of control.

Ms. EE, a 38-year-old woman, recurrently struggled with her therapist about her need for medication. She would press for dosage reduction, despite a good response to sertraline and bupropion and poor response to prior efforts to taper the medication. On questioning, Ms. EE revealed that she felt deeply ashamed about her ongoing need for medication. In fact, she was highly self-critical about her requiring it and felt somehow that taking it suggested she was a bad person.

On exploration, several sources of Ms. EE's shame emerged. At first Ms. EE associated to intense family conflicts, including yelling and occasional physical fighting, between her parents. Ms. EE was fearful that her neighbors could hear these fights, and some comments from her neighbors suggested that they did. Ms. EE's embarrassment about these behaviors was intensified by her parents' dictum that she keep these fights a secret from others.

In the context of these conflicts, Ms. EE saw her mother as particularly out of control. Her yelling would lead to throwing things and sometimes hitting her husband. In addition, her mother's rages would be directed at the patient and her sister. Ms. EE felt something was wrong with her mother, and she associated her own "mental illness"—symptoms of anxiety and depression—with her mother's behavior, even though Ms. EE did not have rages like her mother. However, whenever Ms. EE did feel anger, which was often part of her depression, she would fear that she was going to act just like her mother.

Ms. EE's shame was also related to her mother's critical attacks during her volatile episodes. Her mother would say that Ms. EE was no good or worthless, especially if she made a "mess" by spilling something or if she attempted to defy her mother. Ultimately, this defiance submerged, and Ms. EE became passive–aggressive and self-critical. In particular, her mother blamed Ms. EE for causing her sister's childhood illness through her bad behavior. Thus, Ms. EE saw her symptoms as potentially damaging to others.

Finally, Ms. EE was ashamed that her mother was chronically preoccupied with her health and required constant attention from others to relieve her fears, including multiple doctors' visits. Ms. EE felt that having anxious symptoms made her a burden on others, just as she felt her mother was. These fears emerged in the transference as Ms. EE worried that she was a burden to her therapist.

Ms. EE: I feel very badly that I keep having these symptoms. That I'm not getting any better.

Therapist: Can you say more about what you mean?

Ms. EE: I know you say it doesn't bother you but I don't think you're immune to hearing these troubles every time I come in. (Tearful). I know I must be a burden.

Therapist: First of all, it's not true that you're not getting any better. We've agreed that your depression and anxiety have improved from when you started treatment. I think you are convinced that you are burdensome and that you see it as coming from me.

Ms. EE: Well, it's true I think it's burdensome and you've never said it was, but I find it hard to believe. You're always having to make changes in the medication.

Therapist: I think you see it that way because of your mother's behavior. You and your family found that very difficult to live with. However, your situation is different from hers. For one thing, you have sought help for your problems.

Ms. EE: You know that my mother, despite her own complaints, does not like to hear much about anyone else's problems. Whenever I brought up any kind of issue she would get upset. Maybe that's another reason I expect it so much from you.

Exploring these sources of shame ultimately led to Ms. EE having more tolerance of her symptoms and feeling more comfortable maintaining the medication.

Countertransference Reactions to Compliance Problems

Patients' struggles with compliance are likely to trigger particular types of countertransference reactions for therapists (Book, 1987). Awareness of these issues is helpful in addressing compliance problems when they arise. Although therapists have been trained in a mode of collegial collaboration in psychotherapy, they may revert to a pattern of an authoritative or directive stance that can be more rigid when medication is being discussed or prescribed. As Gutheil noted:

> The same physicians who adopt a receptive, open posture toward their patients' verbal productions may take a rigid, prescriptive stance in relation to drugs, offering direct and specific suggestions, even commands, which they would energetically eschew in the psychotherapeutic interaction. (1982, p. 322)

Although a directive stance is to some degree indicated with medication, therapist rigidity can increase the likelihood that patients' antiauthoritarian tendencies will be triggered.

For example, Book (1987) noted that therapists getting angry at patient noncompliance can trigger several problematic reactions. One such response would be to collude with the patient's noncompliance with a wish that the patient become ill to punish him or her for not following doctor's orders. Another reaction would be an urge to reject or abandon a patient for noncompliance. There may be instances of symptoms being so dangerous and disruptive that a therapist might need to say that treatment without medication is not feasible, but therapists should be alert to the risk that anger at patients could lead them to take this stance when it is not necessary. Finally, a therapist may reproach a patient for not taking the medication according to the prescription. This can cause the patient to be concerned that he is harming the therapist and lead him to comply due to guilty feelings.

A case in which the therapist struggled with countertransference toward the therapist was discussed in chapter 3. Ms. N repeatedly refused to take medication, citing concerns about side effects, particularly fears of bodily damage. She referred to a prior medication trial of fluoxitene in which she experienced agitation that did not resolve until she stopped the drug. The therapist reassured her that the medications being considered would not damage her body and discussed the importance of exploring this concern. In the interim, Ms. N's symptoms intensified with occasional suicidal preoccupations. Therapy appeared to be at a stalemate because the patient's preoccupations were so negative she was not able to step back and consider them with an observing ego. Exploratory efforts to look at the origins of these problems in her intrapsychic conflicts were making little progress.

The therapist became aware of rising frustration and concern, with the countertransference thought: "Why doesn't she just go ahead and take the medication? Why is she defying my suggestions?" He was aware that this thought was unusual for him. In addition, he noticed that he was presenting more dire warnings than usual in his discussion about the medication.

Therapist: Tell me further about your concerns.
Ms. N: Well, I'm worried about the impact of medication on my heart.

Therapist: Can you say more about that?

Ms. N: When my heart starts to beat rapidly, I get worried it's going to stop or that I'm having a heart attack.

Therapist: And how do you feel about your doctors' reassurances about this?

Ms. N: Well, I try to believe them, but the thought is just too scary. I don't want to take any chances with it. I mean doctors can be wrong. They told me my anxiety would go away on the fluoxitene, but it never did.

Therapist: Well, that does happen. In some cases it doesn't get better with fluoxitene. But that's different from the idea that the medication could cause bodily damage. I guess I'm concerned that not taking medication makes therapy very difficult. Your feelings of low self-esteem become so catastrophic that it makes it hard for you to step back and look at them. For instance, you are convinced you are being rejected when you are not.

Ms. N: Well. I'll plan to start them this week.

However, at the next session Ms. N had not yet started the medication, and the therapist was aware of becoming more frustrated.

Therapist: I'm not sure it makes sense to try to continue the therapy if you are not taking the medication.

Ms. N: It sounds like you are very serious about it. But I don't know if I can.

On reviewing this comment, the therapist realized his anger had gotten the better of him. He recognized that this was an extremely unusual statement for him to make and the patient's condition did not really seem so dire. On further reflection, he realized he had become engaged in a power struggle with Ms. N and was angry at her for not following doctor's orders. Discussions about her early conflicts with her father came back to him in a different way. This included the sense not only that he was intrusive and critical but also that he would reject her or abandon her emotionally if she did not follow his edicts. Ms. N reacted with defiance but also felt incapable of performing up to her father's standards academically and frightened about his angry response.

Therapist: I thought about the last session, and I'm not sure it was wise to suggest we might need to end the treatment at this point. What was your experience of what I said?

Ms. N: Well, I was surprised and felt scared and hurt, but I also understand you are very concerned.

Therapist: I guess I had a sense I was becoming like your father, that I was reacting to your struggles by pressuring you to do what I was suggesting.

Ms. N: As you say that, it did feel like that. One thought I had was if you want to pressure me I'll quit first, but then I became very frightened at this prospect. I really need your help.

Therapist: I wonder if this reflects your struggles with your father: You either accepted what he said even if you felt it wasn't right for you or feared losing him if you disagreed.

Ms. N: Yes. That really captures it.

Therapist: Well. I think it's important that we work together to address your fears with the medication rather than repeat the pattern of struggling.

After this discussion, the tensions between the therapist and Ms. N resolved. She tried an alternate SSRI, which also had significant side effects. At that point, Ms. N's fears of the medication as representing and being administered by an intrusive poisonous father emerged. The therapist was able to refer back to the preceding discussion when tensions and fears arose and help the patient separate her transference view of the therapist as father from someone who attempted to understand her anxieties and struggles with medication.

PSYCHOTHERAPY AND MEDICATION AS SYNERGISTIC

Although described before as medication aiding psychotherapy or the reverse, in many instances the two treatments work synergistically. Medication can aid patients in participating in psychotherapy, which can help patients address issues that affect medication treatment. An example of this (as in the case presented next) occurs when effective medication treatment triggers conflicts about success, leading to negative reactions to medication, which can then be explored in psychotherapy. Additionally, medication treatment can be of value in discerning which aspects of the patient's difficulties are based on an obstruction (a biological diathesis) and which are based on resistance (psychological conflict). Medication is necessary to parse out these factors, and psychotherapy is crucial in articulating this delineation.

Difficulty Tolerating Success and Assertiveness From Effective Medication Treatment

Conflicts about assertiveness and success can be exacerbated by effective treatment with medication. In certain instances, depressive symptoms may have averted a conflict surrounding success by diminishing the patient's capacity to achieve certain goals. Relief of symptoms can rapidly allow patients to be more effective and competitive, triggering frightening fantasies in some patients and a need to undo achievement (Freud, 1916).

Ms. FF, a 40-year-old woman, reported recurrent bouts of anxiety, depression, and irritability. In addition to these anxious and depressive symptoms, Ms. FF struggled with inhibitions about achieving success in her profession as a singer. Although she was seen as highly talented, she generally feared singing in public and would stay away from opportunities that would advance her career. Ms. FF responded well to sertraline 100 mg/day. However, she recurrently discontinued the medication, stating that she was becoming concerned about long-term side effects. This pattern persisted despite the fact that her symptoms recurred each time she stopped the medication. In addition, her fears were only temporarily assuaged by the therapist's explanation that there was little evidence of long-term risk of antidepressants, whereas there were significant studies to suggest that persistent anxious and depressive symptoms had adverse effects on health.

In identifying the major factors that inhibited her success, therapist and patient came to focus on Ms. FF's conflicted feelings about her father. Her father was a highly successful lawyer. However, as his success increased, Mr. FF became increasingly self-focused and arrogant. She reported that her father became surrounded by "flatterers" who praised his achievements and did his bidding. When Ms. FF was 10 years old, her father left her mother for a woman he met during his work. She viewed her father's new wife as a schemer with no regard for his children, simply intent on taking advantage of his money and achievement. Her parents became involved in a bitter dispute over many years regarding finances.

Thus, in Ms. FF's mind, success became associated with self-aggrandizement and a disregard for the needs of others. As a means toward success, competitive urges became frightening and conflicted. Increasing effectiveness in her singing along with increased energy and motivation to pursue auditions deriving from antidepressant response created a conflict, leading her to discontinue the medication. Identification with her father as successful but hurtful helped to explain how medications could be damaging.

Despite exploration of these factors, Ms. FF continued to struggle with career pursuits and medication compliance. Additional information emerged on an occasion when the session was interrupted by a pharmaceutical sales representative who was seeking a meeting with the therapist. Ms. FF expressed her concern that the therapist might be corrupted by the sales representative into giving misinformation or understating the potential long-term risks of her medication. When the therapist asked about her further thoughts, Ms. FF recalled a case in which her father represented a pharmaceutical company that was accused of withholding negative information about a case. Her father was successful in defending them, an important development in his career. Ms. FF described how they were taken on a special trip to Hawaii by members of the company, who were highly solicitous of her father. She recalled that this trip was a turning point in his increasing focus on his career and success.

Thus, she feared the therapist could be corrupted just as her father was. However, in this instance, she was able to contrast her experience of the therapist, whose integrity and empathic responsiveness were, in her view, beyond reproach, to the problems that her father experienced. She compared the therapist to a number of friends who she felt had achieved and maintained a consistent humanity. Ms. FF was able to consider alternative representations of self and others that would allow her to achieve more. This discussion also led to increased consistency in taking her medication.

Delineating Chemical and Psychological Contributions to Disorders

As noted in prior chapters, interactional models can help therapists and their patients gain a useful perspective on both the origins of symptoms and the potential role of psychotherapy and medication. In these models, chemical contributions to symptoms can intensify negative affects and associated conflicts, and conflicts and inhibitions can trigger or exacerbate a chemically based disorder. Medication intervention, by presumptively affecting the chemical origins of problems, can help to clarify which aspects of the patient's problems are obstruction versus those that are primarily resistance. Patients may find it helpful to become aware of these interactions for the purpose of accepting combined treatment and to gain an understanding of the feelings and symptoms with which they have been struggling.

Ms. GG described becoming depressed at a point when she was quite angry at her husband, who she reported was becoming obese and was not aggressive in earning money. She became increasingly frustrated and despondent, eventually developing symptoms of a major depressive disorder. However, she also felt intensely guilty about her anger at her husband. When the therapist attempted to discuss with her that her guilt seemed out of proportion, given that she did not express anger directly to him, she replied that she deserved this self-scorn because she was a bad wife. She had trouble with the notion that exploring her fantasies would help to understand why she was self-critical because she felt no explanation was needed. A decision was made to proceed with a medication treatment.

As the medication took effect, the intensity of her anger and guilt eased, and she was now able to address the conflicts regarding her husband. Ms. GG learned through her therapy that she had difficulty tolerating her anger at her husband and felt guilty even though she did not address her concerns with him. Vengeful fantasies deriving from early childhood experiences, associated with a sense that she was to blame for chronic fighting between her parents, were usefully linked to the current problems with her husband. In fact, Ms. GG had a history of being self-critical that predated her depression and, in part, derived from an internalization of comments made by her parents that she was worsening their problems.

In this case, medication intervention not only eased the patient's depression, but also helped to differentiate obstruction (catastrophic levels of anger and guilt) from psychological conflict (superego difficulties in tolerating angry feelings). The information also became useful in addressing Ms. GG's puzzlement as to how she had become so frustrated and guilty, when the problems with her husband seemed relatively minor to her. The therapist suggested that the chemically based depression likely exacerbated her degree of frustration and disappointment and also intensified her guilt, making it even more difficult to deal with the psychological conflicts she had about these feelings. Ms. GG felt relieved by her better understanding of the shift in her perceptions.

CONCLUSION

As indicated previously, several factors may contribute to the combined effectiveness of medication and psychotherapy. Medication can aid psychotherapy not only by reducing disruptive symptoms, but also through presenting opportunities to address psychological factors and conflicts triggered through the employment of psychopharmacology. Psychotherapy can help to relieve patients of several possible adverse reactions to medication, including discomfort with side effects, conflicts around assertiveness, struggles with authority, and feelings of shame. Countertransference reactions may be heightened in the treatment of noncompliant patients. Addressing these issues increases the likelihood that patients will comply with their medication regimen. Awareness of these factors alerts the clinician to opportunities to further the synergistic effects of combined treatment.

6

Approaches to Treatment
The Prescribing Therapist

After the psychoanalyst or psychodynamic therapist determines that medication is indicated, a decision needs to be made as to who should prescribe. The nonphysician therapist, by necessity, must refer the patient to a psychiatrist or sometimes an internist. The unique challenges and opportunities of split treatment will be dealt with in chapter 7. In our experience, most psychodynamic clinicians who feel competent prescribing medication choose to do so for those patients treated in psychotherapy and psychoanalysis. This impression is consistent with the survey data of Doidge et al. (2002) that showed 58% of psychoanalysts in the United States prescribing for patients in psychoanalysis. While this has intuitive appeal, the advantages and disadvantages of this arrangement are poorly studied. This preference suggests that the clinician embraces a biopsychosocial model with his patient, an approach that has been eroded by recent trends within psychiatry (Gabbard & Kay, 2001). This holistic approach can reflect an efficient way of working while offering the clinician a unique opportunity of knowing his patient by virtue of cultivating a "doctor–patient" relationship.

However, the data of Gwynn and Roose (2004), previously cited in chapter 4, suggest that pharmacotherapeutic management may suffer for patients in psychoanalysis with candidate analysts, in an apparent devaluation of the prescribing role. It is not known whether the concerns raised by this study are unique to this patient therapist dyad or apply more broadly, but conflicts persist for many analysts in employing medication. Furthermore, therapist preference can be motivated by countertransference anxieties about split treatment. Idealization of the prescribing role, which can also interfere with optimal treatment, is one way of coping with these anxieties.

Given the current state of knowledge, we believe competent combined treatment can be delivered as a split treatment or by one clinician. In this chapter, we will elucidate relevant considerations for optimizing care when the therapist prescribes. We also postulate that the prescribing therapist has a different state of mind when working with his patient compared to the therapist who works in a split treatment. The difference will affect the therapeutic process in a variety of ways, including how transference is elaborated around the therapist's prescribing. In addition, technical issues arise in how to manage the medication competently during the course of psychotherapy or psychoanalysis. We will discuss the role of free association as it affects this assessment. Finally, termination, always considered a significant phase in a psychodynamic or psychoanalytic treatment, is affected if the therapist is the prescriber since patients often require ongoing prophylactic treatment with drugs after successful psychotherapy.

VALUES OF THE ONE-PERSON TREATMENT MODEL

The appeal of the one-person treatment model is simply put by Gabbard and Kay (2001, p. 1958): "The psychiatrist, like any other good physician, treats the whole person." Embracing a holistic approach implicitly expresses an integrative view of mind and brain that the clinician seeks to cultivate with and within his patient. This perspective often needs to be made explicit in a split treatment (by both members of the treatment team) because this arrangement can encourage a falsely dichotomous perspective: The pharmacotherapist treats the patient's brain while the psychotherapist treats his mind. The prescribing therapist, in his effort to engage in total care, expresses the attitude that issues related to the mind–brain are inextricably linked, and interactions between the two will be focused on in the psychotherapy. The utility of this approach is often apparent at the beginning of treatment when integrative efforts on the part of the clinician model for the patient a way of thinking about complex relationships between medication and introspective approaches.

Mr. O, discussed in chapter 4, presented with symptoms of major depression and panic disorder and was terrified of swallowing a pill because it was linked in his mind with the therapist "fucking with [his] brain." This was associatively connected to a conflicted relationship with his father. Initially, psychotherapy was circumscribed in its focus: to understand the quality of the patient's fears so that he would be able to more realistically consider taking medication. The therapist was explicit in his judgment that the patient's symptomatology and degree of impairment strongly warranted consideration of an SSRI trial.

A predominantly negative paternal transference surfaced as the patient recalled feeling inadequate in relation to a father he experienced as narcissistic and domineering. Analysis of this configuration, including the way it expressed passive yearnings for his father's love as well as his projection of his anger onto the father, freed the patient to accept a medication trial, which gave him substantial relief and opened the way to explore similar kinds of dynamics at work and at home.

In treating Mr. O, the therapist's role as prescriber created a seamless way to deal directly with the patient's anxieties around taking medication while introducing him to the therapist's way of working dynamically. It is precisely because patients' psychodynamics reveal themselves when working with medication that the therapist who feels competent will often prefer to manage it. He or she can feel that referring the patient to a psychopharmacologist is unnecessary or unhelpful; it is unnecessary because he or she has the requisite knowledge to prescribe pharmaceuticals and unhelpful in that many psychopharmacologists are not trained or skilled in managing complex aspects of resistance that require psychodynamic skills.

A variation of this pattern, discussed in chapter 3, involves the patient who accepts medication but resists the recommendation for psychotherapy. Because treating the whole person often requires a sequential approach, a clinician's respect for a patient's ambivalence about engaging in therapy while observing the degree of benefit with medication can create a strong therapeutic alliance. The clinician can empathically explore the resistance to talk therapy, if it still seems indicated, after an adequate medication trial. Sometimes, rather than being a manifestation of resistance, a patient's ego functioning is too impaired to engage in the work of therapy. A clinician providing both medication and psychotherapy can provide an efficient and comfortable way to make this assessment.

Mr. HH was a 30-year-old married male referred for treatment with symptoms of major depression characterized by marked rumination, feelings of worthlessness, insomnia, weight loss, and passive suicidal ideation—a state triggered by a job promotion.

Mr. HH: I make partner at my law firm and I fall apart. What should I do?

Therapist: It's an indication of how depressed you are that you feel that you need me to tell you what to do.

Mr. HH: I'm sure if I hadn't made partner I wouldn't have gotten depressed. Though I've always gotten good reviews, I wonder if the promotion was political rather than an affirmation of my capacities. I'm having a crisis of confidence. But I've been ambivalent about being partner from the beginning. The commitment will make associate's work seem easy by comparison. I've resented the long hours I work. I don't know whether I should stay or leave. I'm confused.

Therapist: Right now your thinking is so affected by your depressive illness that I don't think you're in a position to make such an important decision. What I think you should do for the immediate future is to put any definitive decision on hold until you are feeling better. Then we will be in a better position to understand the complex feelings you have about becoming partner.

Two months later—with a robust response to buproprion—the patient felt substantially improved with a remission of his depressive symptoms and the nature of his interaction with the prescribing therapist changed.

Mr. HH: I'm feeling much stronger mentally and physically. When I was depressed, I thought I couldn't do the job and, in fact, I was too depressed to work. Now, I'm back at work and I know I made partner because I'm competent. But I'm just not sure that this is what I want for myself.

Therapist: We will need to take some time to understand what's been driving you and how it is that you feel so burdened by what appears to be an achievement you've been working toward for years. As you are no longer in a deep depression, we can begin to look at this issue together.

Mr. HH: I realize I couldn't think straight when I was so depressed. And I felt motivated more by anxiety or sheer terror than anything else. But I have a gut feeling I took a wrong turn somehow. But I don't feel so frightened to try to figure things out.

As Mr. HH's depressive illness remitted, the therapist shifted his focus from symptomatic improvement to an exploratory approach, not only to understand the trigger of his vulnerability to depression, but also to help Mr. HH to come to a decision about his job. One year into that treatment, Mr. HH came to realize that his competitiveness had taken on a masochistic dimension. This tendency derived from significant guilt over anger toward his father, whose own professional ambitions resulted in frequent absences from the family. Mr. HH subsequently chose a job as an in-house lawyer with fixed hours, while moving more deliberately to create a family and a more relaxed lifestyle—desires that had been thwarted due to his workaholic tendencies.

COUNTERTRANSFERENCE REASONS FOR SELECTING THE ONE-PERSON TREATMENT MODEL

Alongside the consciously held "ideal" reasons to assume the role of the prescribing therapist, there exist a number of countertransference vulnerabilities that can contribute to a problematic defensive idealization of this dual role. The wish to feel powerful and in control of all facets of the patient's care can reflect an underlying feeling of threat from sharing responsibility in a split treatment. Competitive conflicts can be evoked based on insecurities about the power of therapy compared to medication. Narcissistic vulnerabilities can be triggered; the fact that the patient needs medication can in itself threaten the therapist's identity as therapist. This fear can be managed by insisting on assuming the role of prescriber as a way of containing and taming the "adversary." As will be discussed later, a derivative manifestation of this countertransference is that the therapist forgets about the medication once the psychotherapy gets under way.

One potential expression of the prescribing therapist's countertransference involves the use of his prescribing function as an unconscious way to shackle the patient to a psychotherapy he genuinely believes the patient needs. The "package deal" of combined treatment cannot be refused by the patient out of fear of losing the much needed medication.

Two years into a combined treatment, the therapist referred Ms. II, a woman in her 30s with recurrent major depression and mixed character pathology, for consultation due to the experience of a stalemated psychotherapy process. The stagnation had occurred despite a good medication response and an apparent exploration of important psychological issues related to trust and intimacy. The consultant's impression was that the patient's engagement in therapy reflected a submissive and compliant posture rather than a genuine interest in an introspective process.

The therapist realized that his zeal to engage the patient in psychotherapy blinded him to the patient's lack of motivation for change and to the role of a negative transference. The therapist and patient came to understand that she accepted her need for medication, given the concrete relief she felt when taking it. Her fearfulness about relapse led her to participate reluctantly in an exploratory treatment that focused on paranoid, obsessional, and narcissistic aspects to her character. The patient's engagement in psychotherapy was a manifestation of her paranoid pathology (i.e., she feared not getting medication if she asserted her lack of interest). It was only after treatment was split that this anxiety could be more fruitfully explored and resolved, and the patient ultimately decided to receive only medication treatment.

THE STATE OF MIND OF THE PRESCRIBING THERAPIST

Managing all aspects of the patient's care and having ultimate responsibility for the decision-making on both the therapy and medication fronts lead to process considerations that overlap but are distinct from split treatment. Examining the state of mind of the prescribing therapist compared to a therapist conducting a split treatment helps to clarify these differences. Both must shift their listening between objective and intersubjective perspectives and concern themselves with the various psychological meanings of the medicine to the patient. However, while a therapist in a split treatment must be mindful of how a medication-responsive condition is affecting the patient and his or her treatment, the need for vigilance is attenuated because the therapist can reasonably assume that the pharmacotherapist is periodically doing a careful assessment. The system of split care creates a redundancy that provides a safety net for therapist and patient.

The prescribing therapist, without that fallback, must be certain that the pharmacologic care is not neglected and that enactments around the use of medication are kept to a minimum. While split care does not eliminate these possible difficulties, they are diminished because the pharmacotherapist is less entangled in the patient's transferences. The ultimate responsibility for managing the medication's therapeutic and adverse effects falls to the pharmacotherapist. The ways in which the therapist's prescribing function can become a vehicle for enactments will be discussed later.

Prescribing is not a punctate event. From the moment that the therapist prescribes, the patient develops a bimodal relatedness to him or her (Sandberg, 1998). Unlike the split treatment situation, the patient will move between relating to the clinician as psychotherapist exploring his inner life and as psychiatrist providing symptomatic relief with medication. The oscillation on the part of the patient or prescribing therapist into the doctor–patient mode may reflect the evocation of significant transference or countertransference issues, a legitimate need for reassessment of the pharmacology, or both. Among the questions the prescribing therapist must consider are:

Am I in too much of a rush to prescribe more medication at this point?
Am I inadvertently withholding medication because of how I am choosing to formulate the clinical data?
Why is the patient raising the issue of medication at this particular moment?
Is this serving a defensive function or is he trying to draw my attention to something I've not seen?
Am I not attending to medication because I have become so focused on the patient's psychological issues?
Why is it that neither one of us has said anything about medication for so long?

PROCESS CONSIDERATIONS FOR THE PRESCRIBING THERAPIST

The control the therapist assumes by becoming the prescriber is balanced by the added complexity of working as the pharmacotherapist while working with an evolving transference relationship. It is this dual role that defines the unique position of the prescribing therapist. Some authors have argued that the psychotherapist or psychoanalyst is in the best position to determine the correct dose of a medication by virtue of his immersion in his patient's inner life.

In general, unless one is dealing with fast acting anxiolytics or sedative hypnotic agents, onset of action is typically measured over a period of several weeks and the assessment of a drug's effectiveness is measured based on tracking symptoms that can be ascertained in a more or less objective fashion. This type of assessment does not require the frequency of visits in a usual psychotherapy or psychoanalysis, but this frequency can provide additional data about subtly shifting mood, symptoms, and side effects.

In addition, the prescribing therapist has access to data, usually in the midphase, about the impact of the transference on symptoms, which are typically unavailable to the psychopharmacologist. Whereas some authors caution against the use of such data as extraneous or irrelevant to competent medication management, we believe that they often reflect one crucial piece of information that the prescribing therapist is ideally suited to evaluate. Why is this so? All data are ultimately theory bound. Symptoms that are completely stripped of context (i.e., to be "strictly phenomenological" and atheoretical in the spirit of DSM-IV) run the risk of being incompletely understood and mismanaged. This can especially be the case when the patient is in an intensive therapy in which he experiences change as threatening, and there is a defensive pull to a medical model. In these situations, the patient will often complain of depressive or anxious affect and worry about relapse. Two brief vignettes will illustrate this point.

In the third year of an intensive therapy, Mr. JJ, who suffered from recurrent bouts of major depression and panic disorder treated with buproprion and escitalopram, became increasingly conscious of his idealization of his wife as a defense against his anxiety over being full of rage and destructive. These anxieties stemmed from an identification with a father who had been physically and verbally abusive. He was presently angry that she was forcefully pushing to have a second child without respecting the patient's ambivalence. The therapist had also recently observed that Mr. JJ was viewed as the "sick" spouse within the relationship—a position that both enraged and comforted Mr. JJ. His need for psychiatric treatment reassured him that he was weak and not destructive like his father.

Mr. JJ subsequently came in expressing relief that he was able to tell his wife that he *had* been angry with her for not listening to him and, at the same time, he had decided he did want to have a second child. He also told the therapist he realized the degree to which anxiety interfered with his sense of well-being and asked about buspirone, an antianxiety agent he had taken years ago. A DSM-IV assessment revealed only mild anxiety symptoms, circumscribed to the period of talking to his wife in a more direct way than was characteristic for him. The patient's request for additional medication was understood as part of a complex compromise formation at an important point in the therapy. He was able to be more open about his anger only after asserting that he had changed his mind about wanting a second child (i.e., submitting to his wife's desire). While he was made anxious by this situation, there was no clear indication for additional medication.

Mr. KK had a history of major depression and panic disorder and was being medicated with escitalopram and lorazepam (at bedtime). He presented with a recurrence of insomnia of 3 days' duration. He engaged the therapist in a review of the various agents he had tried for sleep as well as a medical discussion as to whether his insomnia was a trait marker of his depressive illness. No other symptoms suggestive of relapse were present. Mr. KK then went on to talk about his excitement about an upcoming trip with his wife but also had "in the back of [his] mind" that he would be unable to get his usual catch-up sleep on the weekend.

This comment brought both therapist and patient back to an aspect of the patient's attitude about sleep that had been only briefly discussed. His mother had had a chronic illness during his adolescence and frequently needed to take to bed. She died when the patient was in college. Mr. KK subsequently developed a gastrointestinal ailment and told himself that unless he made sure he had enough sleep he could get sick. This fantasy, which unconsciously expressed an identification with his mother, affected not only his attitude about sleep but also how competitive he could be in his professional life. Success, seizing life, was unconsciously linked with losing his mother. While it remained possible that some adjustment in his sleep medicine would be indicated, it became increasingly clear that the patient's fantasy of himself as vulnerable to getting sick and dying was a psychological trigger for his periodic insomnia.

In both situations, the prescribing therapist heard the patients' requests for medicine in a dual way: Does this patient need a medication adjustment, as determined in part by symptom assessment? Is there a psychological need being expressed indirectly through the request? Both patients, in stepping out of their comfort zones, became frightened and fleetingly symptomatic. The hypothesis testing that took place within the therapy also conveyed to the patients a way of thinking and understanding that was neither reductionistic nor authoritarian.

The prescribing therapist is also ideally situated to empathically explore acting out around medication. Patients will often express their conflicts by skipping doses of their medicine, forgetting to take their medication on vacation, or forgetting to ask the therapist for a refill. These forms of acting out directly involve the prescribing therapist and must gain expression within the treatment relationship.

Mr. LL was a man in his mid-20s who suffered from chronic major depression and significant social anxiety characterized by avoidance of women.

Mr. LL: I had a wedding to go to this weekend. I wasn't looking forward to it. It's like I'm the only single guy on the planet. People ask me what's up and I feel like a loser. I didn't want to go to the wedding being around all my friends who are either married or about to get married. I was so upset thinking about it that I forgot to take my Wellbutrin for a few days.

Therapist: Your upset could have taken many forms. Why do you think it took the form of forgetting your medicine?

Mr. LL: When I'm depressed I withdraw. I go to bed and sleep. It seems kind of foolish now, but maybe I was trying to escape going to the wedding by trying to get myself depressed.

Therapist: I think that's an important idea. It's as if you were trying to take care of you—to create a situation of withdrawing from a situation you anticipated would be painful to you—by stopping your medicine.

Mr. LL: I think I need to figure out a better way to cope with how unattractive I feel. Stopping my medicine doesn't seem like a very good solution.

While this interaction could have taken place in a split treatment, the prescribing therapist was particularly curious as to why the patient's upset took the particular form it did—as an acting out around the medicine.

The preceding examples illustrate how the bimodal capacity of the prescribing therapist expresses a competence not only in two distinct forms of therapy but also in managing the relationship between the two. This includes maintaining a psychodynamic perspective as it relates to issues around prescribing and realizing that a patient's request for medication can be overdetermined. This capacity, as has been emphasized throughout the book, is crucial when dealing with a patient who views combining modalities as inherently competitive and antagonistic. When a patient in conflict about medication and psychotherapy is in a split treatment, there must be a well coordinated effort on the part of the team to avoid splitting. With the prescribing therapist, the patient's conflict can be interpreted directly because the therapist conveys an integrated and nonreductionistic approach.

Tutter (2006), previously discussed in chapter 4, presents several vignettes of patients in analysis or intensive psychotherapy who are simultaneously being given medication by the therapist/analyst. Working from an object relations perspective, she elucidates the way in which medication takes on different meanings during the course of treatment. In particular, the medication is seen as representing different objects (including the self; objects from the patient's life, including the analyst; or part objects) during different phases of treatment. For example, she describes the case of a patient (Eamon) being treated with an SSRI for depression, who, during the course of an intensive psychotherapy, expressed his conflicted feelings about depending on the analyst through his ambivalence about taking medicine (hence, the medication represented the analyst). At a later time he saw the medication as a link holding the treatment relationship together, evoking the memory of feeling that he was the "glue" that held his parents' marriage together.

While Tutter (2006) notes that such meanings can evolve in a split treatment, the clinical detail in most of the vignettes presented suggests that the analyst's prescribing role can function as a catalyst to evoke meaning. For example, Eamon's dependency conflicts expressed around medication evolved in a regressed transference toward his prescribing therapist. The medication as "glue" was evoked as the patient anticipated a sabbatical from therapy but was reassured that the therapist would have to continue to renew his prescription.

Other vignettes involve patients complaining that a drug suddenly causes side effects or loses efficacy. In all the vignettes, the analyst is seen as skillfully considering the ways in which the patients' turning to discussions about the medicine reflect displaced references to the transference and a crucial vehicle for its elaboration. We believe that the analyst's prescribing function made her particularly curious and open to discovering the complex and varying meanings with which the patients invested the drug, but that her prescribing role also made her more likely to evoke these meanings. While in theory these transformations could become evident with an analyst engaged in a split treatment, it is unlikely that such subtlety would surface with an analyst who is not prescribing. There is an attunement that takes place where the patient grasps the analyst's curiosity about medicine; this, together with the analyst's concrete prescribing responsibility, makes it more likely that this kind of exploration will become part of the treatment.

While the prescribing analyst may find the analytic process furthered by exploring the various meanings with which medication is invested, this is not inevitably the case. Awad (2001), as noted in chapter 4, presents two clinical cases where there was little, if any, reference to the medication beyond refill requests after the initial period of making the recommendation and analyzing the immediate reaction of his patients: "What was remarkable ... was the absence of any reference to the medication ... it seemed to have faded into the background" (p. 273). This experience is not unlike that of others who note that effective pharmacology can facilitate the psychotherapeutic process without the meaning of medication occupying a significant aspect of the analysis per se (Wylie & Wylie, 1995).

Tutter and Awad reveal two poles on the continuum of good analytic work with patients on medication. For some patients, or perhaps some dyads, the prescribing function will be a stimulus for the elaboration of particular conflicts and fantasies, the analysis of which will deepen the therapeutic process. For others, competent combined treatment can manifest as a freeing up of an obstructed process with particular meanings of medicine occupying a minor part of the treatment. These clinical possibilities, however varied, reflect a relatively uncomplicated scenario: Medication is effective, side effects are not prominent, and problematic enactments are avoided. Often, the reality of clinical work forces the clinician to confront more complex situations.

ENACTMENTS AND THE PRESCRIBING THERAPIST

Enactments express the unconscious emergence of a patient's conflicts in the form of action between patient and therapist. It is generally agreed that enactments are an inevitable, even constant, aspect of analytic work, though opinions differ as to whether the therapist should be vigilant to keep enactments to a minimum (Steiner, 2006) or whether such vigilance risks losing essential grist for the therapeutic mill (Levenson, 2006). The therapist's prescribing can be a vehicle for enactments. Examples include introducing medication when it is not indicated or withholding medication when it is.

While enactments will also occur when medication has been appropriately prescribed (for example, a depressed patient is given an antidepressant and elaborates a fantasy of impregnation by the therapist), we focus here on the vulnerability of the prescribing therapist to enactment due to countertransference issues. In a split treatment, the presence of a pharmacotherapist who is less entangled in the patient's transference and who typically focuses on objective criteria for medicating functions as a safeguard. It can be challenging for the prescribing therapist to maintain such an objective focus under the sway of his countertransference. Two recent examples in the literature illustrate these issues.

Greene (2001) presented a treatment of a woman he analyzed that involved "experiments" with fluoxetine. Among the relevant factors for this discussion are: the patient presented with symptoms of atypical depression while the initial diagnostic impression was phobic neurosis and hysterical personality; the patient requested antidepressant treatment while the analyst recommended psychoanalysis and indicated his opposition to the use of medication in analysis; while the patient periodically expressed depressive content ("sailing on a sea of depression," "falling into a black hole") fluoxetine was never introduced to treat depressive symptoms.

The analyst acquiesced to the patient's request to try fluoxetine for weight loss despite the fact that the patient had lost (and regained) 30 pounds at the beginning of treatment (off medication) and fluoxetine is not indicated for the treatment of obesity. Fantasies of seduction and impregnation ensued along with reconstructions of a traumatic and incestuous childhood experience with an older brother. Transient weight loss during the "experiment" of fluoxetine treatment resembled the patient's weight loss at the beginning of the analysis, cluing both patient and analyst in to the importance of the medication as a vehicle for an enactment of important events/fantasies from childhood.

Greene concluded, "It seems likely that a patient's insistence on the analyst's prescribing suggests a specific transference reenactment is about to occur, a reenactment that is more important than the medication per se" (p. 626). He further views his case as refuting "the claims of analysts who have advocated a bimodal therapy on the assumption that many ... patients have two diseases" (p. 627). We suggest that while the analyst and patient learned from the enactment, such events do not inevitably further the therapeutic process. Also, while the author uses the case to refute the utility of a bimodal approach, we believe the analyst must consider whether medication is actually indicated. The analyst did not accept and did not properly assess the patient for the presence of a second disease.

Enactments can also be expressed by the nonintroduction of medication. Abel-Horowitz (1998) describes, with unusual candor, his work as a candidate analyst with a male patient while his supervisor strongly discouraged the use of medication. The patient, who had previously been prescribed medication for several months when first meeting the analyst, escalated his requests/demands for fluoxetine coincident with his involvement in analysis. Months went by with the patient complaining of feeling increasingly depressed and anxious and with the analyst maintaining an interpretive focus within the transference and recommending that the patient intensify his analysis rather than begin medication. Finally, when the patient presented with suicidal ideation, weight loss, and angina, the analyst capitulated and prescribed fluoxetine with immediate relief for the patient, suggesting that a sadomasochistic encounter was a source of stress for the patient.

Abel-Horowitz observed, "The evidence mounted that the patient's perceived need for medication masked and expressed a deeper need to engage me sadomasochistically" (1998, p. 687). He also postulated that his reluctance to prescribe medication inevitably shaped the patient's resistance, and this reluctance was linked to anxieties around analytic identity formation and educational progression. While the analyst noted his patient's "perceived need" for medication, the clinical report made clear that the patient had a depressive syndrome. The particular tensions around developing and displaying an analytic sensibility probably contributed to the analyst formulating that a sadomasochistic tendency was primary relative to the depressive illness. Such tendencies are often exacerbated by depressive illness and their presence, if accentuated by a mood disorder, may be reduced to a manageable and analyzable intensity when the mood disorder is treated psychopharmacologically.

FREE ASSOCIATION AND COMBINED TREATMENT

Perhaps the greatest challenge for the prescribing therapist is the ongoing assessment and management of the pharmacologic aspect of the treatment. This is distinct from the analyst/therapist maintaining a curiosity about the psychological meaning of the medication for the patient. The systematic assessment of doses, symptoms, and side effects is in stark contrast to the technique of free association. Most dynamic clinicians encourage the patient to speak freely and openly about what comes to mind without imposing an agenda. While free association may give the dynamic therapist deeper insights into various unconscious meanings medication has for the patient, no compelling argument can be made that free association is either necessary or sufficient for competent medication management.

Roose and Johannet (1998) discuss how the importance of free association historically functioned as a resistance for analysts using medication; more recently, Cabaniss and Roose (2005) have raised concerns as to how the reliance on free association as an essential dimension of dynamic work can hinder pharmacologic management. While this concern may be especially significant with psychoanalysis, we believe that all dynamic psychotherapists must confront the tendency to adhere to free association as a potential inhibitor of appropriate psychopharmacologic management.

In fact, once a patient begins treatment in a combined modality, the therapist must periodically assess what adjustments in doses of medicine are necessary and monitor the occurrence of side effects. Early in treatment, the patient's motivation for symptomatic relief will often lead him to discuss issues related to medication. However, as treatment progresses, these considerations tend to recede because symptoms usually improve and a successful induction into an insight-oriented process tends to move the patient from the more surface aspects of his experience to a curiosity about deeper motivations. Medication management, especially if it is a significant source of anxiety for the patient, can be experienced as disruptive or intrusive.

Mr. MM began treatment with his current therapist on a complex regimen that included sertraline, clonazepam, and olanzapine after he relocated from another city. His history was notable for repeated bouts of major depression since late adolescence. Olanzapine, an atypical psychotic, had been very helpful for chronic insomnia and may have played a role in stabilizing his mood. He had never been psychotic or manic. While he did not gain significant weight on the drug, his lipid profile was elevated—a side effect reported with this medication. The therapist was concerned about these side effects and felt the patient should consider alternate agents.

Therapist: I notice that each time I bring up my concerns about your continuing to take olanzapine, you express annoyance with me.

Mr. MM: That's because it seems to me it's your agenda, not mine. I'm very busy and stressed at work and I don't want to rock the boat by considering making any changes with the medicine.

Therapist: I realize that you have been deeply depressed in the past and neither one of us wants you to relapse. You will probably need medication for the rest of your life. However, I am not sure if your prior doctor talked to you about the potential risks of olanzapine or if you feel so frightened to get depressed again that you don't want to even talk about the issues related to its use.

Mr. MM: I realize that I frequently tell you this isn't a good time to talk about it. There's always something stressful going on. But I do think I want to put off the discussion because I'm afraid of making any change.

Therapist: I think it's important you can identify this tendency. At the same time, I think we need to set aside time to review the potential risks of tardive dyskinesia and metabolic issues related to the medicine so that you are fully informed and can make a decision based on adequate information.

Mr. MM: I agree that we should decide on a time to discuss this—kind of like scheduling an appointment to deal with the medication. Otherwise, I'll keep running from the issue. And besides it's not like what we're talking about (apart from the medication) is unimportant. I've been working hard in the therapy and I don't want to lose the continuity of our discussions.

Are there times when an assessment is unnecessary outside of the patient's free associations? If the clinician finds the data for responsible medication management surfacing as a spontaneous part of the patient's free associations, then he need not artificially interrupt the flow of associations. In our experience, this is a rare occurrence. Furthermore, because of the sway of transference, the clinician cannot assume that because a patient is not complaining about new symptoms or side effects that they are not present.

Ms. NN was a 45-year-old single woman with a long history of recurrent depression treated with venlafaxine. She was in a twice-weekly psychotherapy in an effort to help her with relationship issues characterized by a desire to please others at her own expense. The therapist, maintaining a psychotherapeutic perspective, consistently focused on how her unhappiness seemed related to a predictable pattern of bending over backward to please others, as if that would give her the love and approval she craved, while she was inevitably disappointed and angry. This behavior recapitulated an important pattern from her childhood. At one point, Ms. NN commented on how tired she was and that she had spent most of the weekend in bed. The therapist considered whether the patient had a recurrent depressive syndrome.

It was only upon direct questioning that Ms. NN acknowledged having had suicidal ideation over a period of a couple weeks—something that surprised the therapist. In hindsight, he realized that the patient's core character problem manifested itself in the transference in the form of not spontaneously letting the therapist know about her degree of hopelessness and despair. Not revealing the depth of her emotional pain was a way to try to take care of the therapist (by not burdening him) while fearing that her misery would provoke rejection. The patient and therapist became aware of the need for increased attention to her depressive symptoms and to her tendency to withdraw from the very person whose help she craved.

RESIDUAL MOOD SYMPTOMS OR CHARACTER?

The discussion about free association relates to another complex aspect of combined treatment. It is often unclear when listening to clinical material whether one is dealing with character pathology, residual mood symptoms, or some admixture. The clinician can work for a period of time psychotherapeutically and, depending on the response of the patient, may find himself rethinking his formulation. Reconsidering medication can reflect a countertransference on the part of the clinician who is tired or angry with a patient who seems entrenched in his misery.

Countertransference can also manifest itself when one works for prolonged periods of time in psychotherapy, overlooking the possibility that residual mood symptoms have created an obstruction to the therapeutic process (Wylie & Wylie, 1995). Split treatment creates its own complications because either member or both members of the treatment team can be burdened by countertransference attitudes that interfere with an optimal kind of hypothesis testing. However, for the therapist providing combined treatment, the specific countertransferences involve the simultaneous risks of avoiding drug considerations or pursuing them too aggressively.

Dr. OO, a mental health professional, had a long history of dysthymia along with significant masochistic pathology. She accepted a trial of buproprion that gave her substantial benefit, though she continued to be downcast and pessimistic, with low self-esteem, characterized by a feeling of being unlovable and unloving. These feelings occurred in the setting of substantial early trauma that was symbolically recapitulated when her engagement broke up. After a year of psychotherapy, and another disappointment in a romantic relationship, the therapist entertained the idea that a trial of augmenting with escitalopram might be helpful. The patient was reluctant.

Dr. OO: Like I said, I'm borderline (said pejoratively). I have affective instability. This guy breaks up with me and I'm devastated. It's only been 3 weeks. They say that it takes half the time to get over someone as the time you've gone out, so maybe I won't feel so low over the next 3 weeks—that would be half the time we dated.

Therapist: You're familiar with the typical symptoms of clinical depression. Are other symptoms present?

Dr. OO: My sleep is interrupted the way it always is. I've been distracted but that's understandable because this guy dumped me. But I went out over the weekend with my friends and a couple guys talked to me and I felt happy. I'm not particularly hopeful about my circumstance but that's nothing new and my self-esteem—it's never very good.

Therapist: You tend to view yourself harshly and labeling yourself "borderline" is an example of that. I don't think it is possible to know for sure what we are dealing with since what we are talking about can be viewed in different ways. Your mood is reactive but that doesn't mean you're not depressed. And of course your sleep difficulties have also been a frequent feature of your depressive illness. I think the best we can do is to consider the pros and cons of a medication trial while acknowledging that we can't know for certain if it will help unless we decide to try.

Dr. OO: I'll think about it some more. Maybe I will see how I feel over the next week. But I still think I have borderline pathology.

Therapist: I think your insistence on being borderline, without denying your difficulties in getting close to people, is an expression of a chronic low-grade depression. You have difficulty being benevolent with yourself and your training has become a weapon that you now use against yourself.

In this vignette, the therapist, after multiple prior efforts at trying to engage the patient in a more aggressive medication trial, became more pointed in addressing the resistance. There had been a long period of psychotherapeutic work that produced limited gains, leading the therapist to question whether more time, an intensification of treatment, a different kind of psychotherapy, or a medication trial was needed. These questions were raised as part of the therapy process.

While the vignette suggests that the patient and therapist had competing views of how to understand what was going on, the patient's perspective—one that placed an emphasis on character—also reflected a consideration entertained by the therapist. However, as he shifted his assessment to that of the mood disorder being partially treated, his interpretive focus shifted. This was evident in how he interpreted her lament that she was borderline as evidence of a depressive trait rather than as a sign of masochism.

SIDE EFFECTS AND THE PRESCRIBING THERAPIST

In chapter 5, we discussed the usefulness of a psychotherapeutic approach in helping patients deal with side effects and their impact on the clinical situation. The prescribing therapist may be particularly vulnerable to countertransference reactions that compromise care. Writing for psychoanalysts and focusing primarily on SSRIs, Glick and Roose (2006) suggest an interwoven series of countertransference fantasies that can be evoked when patients experience side effects. Of particular significance are fantasies of forbidden pleasures and boundary violations (e.g., the act of prescribing may be experienced as an erotically charged penetration of the patient). Fantasies of having harmed the patient can be kindled by the reality of having prescribed a drug that has caused a side effect. This can create blind spots in clinical management as suggested by the following vignette reported by the authors.

Two years into the analysis of a young woman described as chronically depressed and masochistic, the analyst realized she had unconsciously withheld medication from the patient in an effort to be a new curative object. An antidepressant was subsequently prescribed with a positive effect on mood and increased socialization. However, "the patient quietly hinted that her formerly strong and pleasurable, and very private masturbatory sexual feelings were quite dampened" (p. 757). The analyst initially responded by acknowledging this was a side effect; it could improve over time or the medication could be changed. The patient subsequently stopped dating and considered stopping the medication.

The analyst then shifted the interpretive focus to the patient's (sado)masochistic motivation to be victorious over the analyst, expressed by the wish to stop the medication. When the patient's request to discontinue the medication resurfaced later (now with her acknowledging feeling better), the analyst, aware of the high risk of relapse off medication, preempted the premature discontinuation of the medication via interpretation and "hence avoided enacting another masochistic transference reaction (p. 757)." Since no further discussion of the sexual side effect is noted, the reader is left wondering if the analyst, in an effort to avoid one masochistic scenario (preventing relapse into depression), had inadvertently enacted another (compelling the analysand to stay on a drug that diminished her libido).

The management of drug side effects can be complex for nontransferential reasons. There are no easy remedies for many side effects and patient and pharmacotherapist will often have to engage in a risk-benefit assessment to determine the best way to intervene. When an evolving transference (and vulnerability to countertransference) is added to the mix, one can see opportunities and pitfalls when the therapist is also responsible for having to make potentially difficult treatment decisions.

In the preceding scenario, the analyst may have been more focused on a facet of the clinical situation that was easier to manage. That is, viewing the patient's masochism reflected in the urge to stop medication led to a straightforward recommendation that she stay on the medicine. Had the focus been on the patient's masochism being expressed by staying on a drug that impaired her libido, the pharmacologic steps would have been less clear. In addition, the fact that the analyst had a role in creating the side effect would also have come into the analysis. This vignette highlights that in an intensive therapy the patient's associations will be affected by her transference to the analyst. The quiet hint of impaired libido, as can best be discerned by the clinical report, became silent. The therapist/analyst cannot assume that because the patient has not complained of a side effect that one does not exist.

While direct questioning about side effects increases the likelihood of discovering them, it is naive to think that a patient's defensive activity will be overcome by this approach. Patients can minimize problematic side effects out of a fear of angering the therapist or because the side effect feels too embarrassing to discuss. Sometimes complaints about side effects will surface during the course of treatment and reveal something important about the state of the transference.

Ms. PP was a single woman in her mid-40s who presented with a major depression after her brother died of cancer. An SSRI was prescribed with good benefit. Having lost her mother to alcoholism when she was a child, the patient tended to function in a maternal role with her large extended family. She had not dated in many years. Toward the latter part of the first year of a twice weekly psychotherapy, Ms. PP revealed that the medication had dampened her libido. This came as a surprise to the therapist because the patient had been so vocal about being uninterested in a romantic relationship.

In fact, the patient had a very active fantasy life—one that was embarrassing, shameful, and exciting. The SSRI had markedly diminished her capacity for erotic fantasy and sexual arousal. The transference at the time of this revelation had erotic overtones of which the therapist was unaware. Exploration revealed that the patient was trying to compel the therapist to express dissatisfaction with her for not finding a job more quickly. This wish to be punished was associatively linked to her erotic life that centered on a beating fantasy by a parental authority figure.

A further associative link was that she had been a "bad girl" for not disclosing anything about her sexual fantasy life. She was both fearful and desirous of displeasing the therapist to provoke punishment. This process opened the door to a discussion about her conflicted sexual life; complaining about the side effect was an expression of a deepening therapeutic process that both excited and frightened her. Coincident with this exploration, the patient was switched to buproprion (a drug much less likely to cause sexual side effects).

THE PRESCRIBING THERAPIST AND TERMINATION

A survey by Yang et al. (2004) found that a significant number of patients treated in analysis with medication continue in pharmacologic treatment with the analyst once the treatment ends. The evidence-based view that most major psychiatric illnesses are chronic in nature supports the clinical wisdom of long-term medication prophylaxis for many patients. It is not clear how the ongoing presence of the therapist as pharmacotherapist affects the experience of termination. We are not aware of any evidence to suggest that the analytic outcome in such cases is suboptimal, though the possibility exists that the ongoing relationship to the analyst as pharmacotherapist could be used defensively to fend off a deeper process of mourning.

The analyst as a real person whose "realness" has therapeutic weight is increasingly accepted among clinicians from different theoretical persuasions. Supportive measures are a frequent aspect of less intensive psychotherapies. An enduring pharmacotherapeutic relationship can be seen as extending the supportive, "real" role of the therapist or analyst. However real the ongoing contact is for the patient, the therapist will no longer be in the patient's life in the same way, as both the quality and frequency of contact change. The awareness of these realities facilitates the process of mourning.

Mr. O (previously discussed in chapter 4) was ending a successful 2-year psychotherapy for chronic anxiety and depression while continuing with an SSRI as a maintenance treatment. During the course of treatment he had become increasingly comfortable asserting himself at work and within his marriage and felt more manly as he took the initiative to have a period of couple's therapy to improve his sex life with his wife. The anxiety of being "fucked with"—an early transference manifestation—had given way to feeling more potent. In the weeks prior to termination he developed a recurrence of his panic symptoms that led him to reconsider whether ending treatment was premature.

Mr. O: This may not be a good time to stop coming. My anxiety seems to have come back. This is what brought me here in the first place.

Therapist: We have been able to see how you've become so much more comfortable asserting yourself at work and with your wife. Perhaps you're anxious because it's hard for you to say good-bye to me and to assert that you don't need to depend on me as you have in the past.

Mr. O: Am I all better? Am I going to be able to do okay without seeing you so frequently? I know when I first came to see you I feared you were fucking with my brain. I've been helped a lot but I guess if I were all better I wouldn't need medicine.

Therapist: Your ability to accept medicine reflects one way in which you have gotten better. You were able to overcome your terror of being hurt and to do what was necessary to feel better. While you worry that you're fragile, I think that taking charge of your life and feeling more manly, in relation to me, causes you anxiety—as if a part of you feels that you should stay to feel dependent on me.

Mr. O: You've consistently taken the position that I am a man who is fearful of assuming my place in the world as opposed to a child who's not capable of functioning. I've appreciated that but it still feels kind of scary. And while I've complained at times about how I've felt depending on you, I'll miss these sessions because I know you've been in my corner.

In subsequent visits that occurred at monthly and then bimonthly intervals, the patient at first expressed anxiety and some sense of awkwardness about how to relate to his now former therapist. The meetings were semistructured, intended to assess his overall functioning. The patient's ongoing consolidation of the psychotherapeutic work was evident during these meetings with further improvements in his work and home life and enhanced self-esteem. The medication also became integrated as a fact of life. The therapist's experience was of a termination process that had been helpful to the patient but also attenuated in its intensity (for both participants) because of the ongoing relationship.

Suggestions for Minimizing Risks When Functioning as the Prescribing Therapist

There are a number of ways in which the prescribing therapist can minimize the risks and make prescribing more effective:

- Monitor countertransference. Countertransference problems can manifest themselves in a variety of ways. The therapist can be hasty in prescribing during difficult stretches of the therapy or can withhold medication in order to have the treatment be a more "pure" psychotherapy. The therapist should be alert to enactments that occur with medication management.
- The therapist must occasionally interrupt free association to obtain the necessary data for ongoing assessment and management. He should periodically consider what he actually knows, by virtue of the free associative process, about the target symptoms for which the patient receives medication. Balancing the focus on the patient's subjective experience with the need to elicit data for adequate medication management can be a complex task for the therapist.
- Know limitations. There will be times when combining treatment will be too difficult for a given analyst. For example, patients often do not respond to an initial trial of medication or require various combinations to bring about remission. Side effects can be significant. Medication refractory patients often require less studied interventions to improve. Many patients have comorbid medical illnesses requiring additional medication, which can have psychological effects as well as potentially serious interactions with psychotropic

drugs. The therapist may have difficulty managing the medication in these complex situations and may require expert psychopharmacological assistance. At times, the incursion of the medical aspects of treatment can overwhelm the psychotherapy and treatment needs to be split. The clinician benefits from knowing the limits of his expertise with regard to psychopharmacology as well as the acceptable and tolerable incursions of pharmacotherapy into the psychotherapy relationship.

CONCLUDING COMMENTS

The prescribing therapist epitomizes the good physician in his effort to treat the whole patient. The skill set for this combined function goes beyond a dual capacity to engage in psychotherapy and prescribe medication. In this chapter, we have attempted to show that a dynamic relationship exists in the mind of the therapist as he attempts to deliver both types of treatment competently and empathically. As an ideal, the treatment can benefit from an enriched process evoked in relation to the therapist's prescribing function. At the same time, the exploratory process must take place alongside responsible medication management, not at its expense. An awareness of the risks of enactment, the need to interrupt free association for systematic assessment, and technical problems emanating from side effects increases the likelihood that the psychiatrist will be effective in providing combined treatment.

7

Split Treatment

Split treatment is a term for therapeutic intervention involving a therapist providing psychotherapy and a psychiatrist (or occasionally other medical practitioners) prescribing medication. This type of treatment has been increasingly frequent as safer medications and use of medication for a broader range of syndromes have led to more requests by therapists for psychopharmacologic evaluation and intervention. In addition, insurance and managed care programs have pressured patients toward pursuing a typically less expensive psychotherapy by a nonpsychiatrist, alongside a less frequent psychopharmacological visit. These "treatment triangles" can allow for the synergistic collaboration of practitioners and treatments with successful relief of patients' symptoms and conflicts. However, these arrangements also have the potential for transference and countertransference problems and conflicts between practitioners that can disrupt effective treatments.

Therapists who are not licensed to prescribe medication require a physician for psychopharmacological intervention. Although many psychiatrists who are psychotherapists act as the psychopharmacologist, some elect, for a variety of reasons, to have another psychiatrist perform the psychopharmacological evaluation and treatment. One basis for this choice is a lack of adequate knowledge about or experience with medication. Another concern is that medication interventions will disrupt the psychotherapeutic or psychoanalytic process (Kelly, 1998).

POTENTIAL CONFLICTS IN TREATMENT TRIANGLES

Gould and Busch (1998) and Busch and Gould (1993) described potential areas of conflict between the practitioners as including underlying competitive pressures, frustration with the other practitioner's approach in a difficult case, differing theoretical and clinical conceptualizations of the nature of the patient's illness, and proprietary feelings toward the patient. Competitive pressures can develop from perceived status issues and power differential between practitioners with different degrees. In addition, tensions can arise about "sharing" a patient deriving from economic concerns. For instance, some patients may state that for financial reasons they need to cut back on the frequency of one or the other treatment. Additionally, therapists may develop concerns about another clinician "stealing" a patient. Although sometimes well intentioned (one practitioner believing that the patient can benefit better through work with him or her alone), competitive, economic, and countertransference factors are often active, and it is not unusual for this type of treatment to develop further problems.

For instance, a psychiatrist was using medication and psychotherapy to treat a complex female patient in her early 50s who had been traumatized by the suicide of her mother when she was an adolescent and by a recent separation from her husband. Ms. QQ had received a series of medication trials, but only responded to an MAO inhibitor, phenelzine. After her husband announced that he wanted to leave her, he reported that he would consider marital therapy. The psychiatrist referred them to a couples' therapist. After several sessions, however, it was clear that the husband was intent on leaving and would not reconsider.

At this point, the couples' therapist suggested that Ms. QQ should switch to individual therapy with her because she felt that a woman would help make up for the deficit in maternal care that the patient had received. In addition, her sense was that the patient was too angry with men to make progress with the psychiatrist. The psychiatrist did not feel these factors were central, believing that the patient had to cope with abandonment fears and threats she experienced from others' narcissistic preoccupations independently of the therapist with whom she was working. Both her mother and husband were focused on their appearance and status, with little attention to the patient's needs. In addition, Ms. QQ was concerned about how her depression was affecting her daughter and feared repeating and unconsciously reenacting her mother's behavior with her.

It emerged, however, that the marital therapist had already addressed her view with the patient and that Ms. QQ felt similarly that the couples' therapist was a better "match." The psychiatrist was frustrated with the therapist for having discussed this with the patient prior to addressing it with him. However, given that the patient already favored this plan and considering the possibility that this alternative "match" may be of value, he acceded to the plan.

For a time the new therapy seemed to proceed very well. Ms. QQ appeared to be feeling "held" by the therapist, who attempted to help the patient understand her pull toward involvement with narcissistic others and help her establish a social life not involving the husband. She also met with the patient and daughter and was able to point out Ms. QQ's criticalness and self-preoccupation when with her daughter. However, Ms. QQ soon began to complain about the therapist when she came to her psychiatrist for medication sessions. She focused on her rigidity, including being charged for missed sessions and the therapist's unwillingness to adjust the frequency from twice to once weekly as the patient was attempting to develop a more active social life. The psychiatrist was aware of urges to say, "I told you so," but attempted to address Ms. QQ's concerns in his own sessions and with the therapist. However, the patient became increasingly frustrated and terminated the relationship with the therapist, returning to therapy with the psychiatrist.

As will be described later, various factors can contribute to the "splitting" of a treatment triangle. Problems could have been avoided in this case by a greater discussion of options before the marital therapist spoke with the patient. Maintenance of a "triadic therapeutic alliance," described by Kahn (1991), is a useful model in addressing problems that can arise in a treatment triangle. In this conception, therapist and psychopharmacologist should be working in tandem with a goal of helping the patient. The triadic therapeutic alliance includes mutual respect among therapist, pharmacotherapist, and patient for the interventions being employed. In addition, thoughtful discussions of problems and disagreements and how to approach them can be crucial for maintaining the alliance. In Kahn's view, a positive triadic therapeutic alliance could correlate with treatment outcome just as a therapeutic alliance between the patient and therapist has been found to in studies.

Transference and Countertransference Issues

Gould and Busch (1998) described transference and countertransference issues that typically develop in treatment triangles. A common transference theme at the time of initial consultation, which can be present consciously or unconsciously, is that the therapist is rejecting the patient or feels the patient is too sick for psychotherapy alone. In addition to exploring these feelings if they should arise, the therapist should provide proper psychoeducation about the role and function of the psychopharmacologist and the fact that psychotherapy will continue as it had previously.

Additionally, patients can idealize the psychopharmacologist following the rapid relief of symptoms that often occurs with medication. This can be associated with a devaluation of the therapist for not having suggested medication sooner or for not being able to prescribe the helpful medication. These feelings can be exacerbated by the more directive and interventive style of the psychopharmacologist, with a sense that the therapist has been withholding by comparison. Idealization of the psychopharmacologist and medication can shift, however, when patients realize that the medication is not a "cure-all," such as when symptoms recur or there are persistent side effects. At that point, devaluation of the psychopharmacologist and medication becomes a possibility.

Idealization of the medication can serve as a basis for resistance to addressing more complex negative feelings toward the therapist. Patients can "explain" frustration at the therapist by focusing on the greater directiveness of the psychopharmacologist and the effectiveness of the medication. Therefore, transference longings and deprivations with the less "gratifying" psychotherapist can be avoided. Sometimes this may require more direct explanations of the functions and role of the psychotherapist and psychopharmacologist. Under these circumstances, support for the psychotherapy by the psychopharmacologist may be crucial to avoid a disruption in the treatment.

Countertransference can affect the reactions to a consultation for medication evaluation. Psychotherapists can feel inadequate due to their inability to prescribe medication or may feel reluctant to expose their psychotherapeutic work to another practitioner. In addition, they can feel a lack of control with regard to management of the case and become concerned that the patient's care may be mishandled. Both practitioners can be susceptible to colluding with the patient in criticisms toward the other practitioner, such as the urge the psychiatrist felt in the case of Ms. QQ earlier. The patient may tell the psychopharmacologist that "I'm really not getting anywhere in therapy" or report to the therapist that "the psychopharmacologist does not really get me. He's just interested in my symptoms." Clinicians can be drawn in by patients' comments due to competitive, narcissistic, or economic pressures. As noted before, clinicians should be alert to avoiding these pitfalls and address patients' concerns with the other practitioner.

Role Diffusion

Role diffusion can also create complications in a split treatment case. For instance, a therapist may make recommendations to the patient about changes in medication without discussing it with the therapist. Similarly, a psychopharmacologist, particularly if he is also a psychoanalyst, may be tempted to make interpretations or clarifications to the patient regarding conflicts or other psychotherapeutic interventions or suggestions. Sometimes these comments can be helpful or benign, but at other points they may involve a wish to be the therapist or undermine the therapist's position. As with other issues, the collaborative arrangement between the practitioners is a factor: In some therapeutic triangles, the clinicians may not have a problem with the other clinician giving input, whereas others may feel intruded upon or undermined. In either case, if clinicians are commenting to the patient about the other's interventions, they should monitor their motives. Ultimately, the other practitioner should be informed about the suggestion to avoid a sense of collusion between the patient and that practitioner.

For instance, a patient, Ms. RR, contacted the psychopharmacologist after a therapy session stating that the therapist had suggested an increase in her dose of Concerta for ADD. The patient had forgotten that she had tried this dose before and had not reacted well. Although the psychopharmacologist was aware of some irritation about the therapist speaking directly to the patient about this, he felt the therapist generally had a good sense of the patient's symptoms and medication needs. He contacted the therapist and discussed the medication issue, and then added in that, in general, he preferred the therapist speak directly with him when suggesting medication changes.

Differing Theoretical and Clinical Models

Differing theoretical and clinical views of patients can create a disruption in a treatment triangle. Most typically this will occur in the context of a psychiatrist viewing a patient's symptoms as chemically related and treatable with medication changes, whereas the therapist may identify the symptoms as psychologically based with the most appropriate intervention being psychotherapeutic. Split treatment is susceptible, therefore, to practitioners employing a two-illness model, disputing the interaction between biology and psychology. Malin (1998) attributes these problems to the intrusion of metatheories into clinical work; metatheories, such as intrapsychic conflict underlying neurosis or the biochemical basis of symptoms, can obscure consideration of other contributors or approaches to the patient's problems.

For instance, in a case described by Gould and Busch (1998), a psychoanalyst's metapsychological theories led him to view psychopharmacological interventions as secondary or unnecessary. The patient's depression initially responded to the antidepressant prescribed by a consulting psychopharmacologist. After tapering the medication, however, the patient suffered a recurrence, and the psychopharmacologist recommended the medication be restarted. The psychotherapist, however, felt that because he now understood what was occurring psychodynamically with the patient's depression, medication was not needed. The persistence of symptoms, as well as psychoeducation by the psychopharmacologist, led the psychotherapist to reconsider his stance.

A similar error could be made by a psychopharmacologist, who detects a pattern of symptoms consistent with a syndrome that is medication responsive and concludes that psychotherapy is a needless intervention. An understanding of interactional models of psychopharmacology and psychotherapy, described in chapter 2, can be crucial in easing split treatment conflicts stemming from differing theoretical and clinical perspectives.

Gender Issues

Due to the increasing presence of women in the mental health field, the combination of a female psychotherapist with a male psychopharmacologist occurs frequently. Gender-related transferences will be likely to arise in the setting of psychopharmacological consultation. For example, as noted by Gould and Busch (1998), a male patient can avoid frightening erotic longings for the female therapist by idealizing a male psychiatrist. The female patient may view the male psychopharmacologist as a rescuer from an intense maternal transference or as an object for oedipally based competitive feelings with the therapist. Gender-based reactions will also occur with a male therapist and female psychopharmacologist. Clinicians should be alert to how these transference fantasies affect the split treatment.

COMMUNICATION BETWEEN PRACTITIONERS

As can be noted from the discussion thus far, we recommend communication between the psychopharmacologist and psychotherapist regarding a number of issues. However, employing an "abstinent" model in treating a patient with medication, Kelly (1998) suggested minimal communication. As noted in chapter 3, according to Kelly, a psychoanalyst employing the "abstinent" model would avoid prescribing medication because he is employing a nonanalytic approach that disrupts abstinence. Even if the analyst uses an "interventionist" model and prescribes the medication, he should attempt to remain neutral (e.g., avoid taking sides in the patient's decision).

In Kelly's view, the "abstinent" and "neutral" psychoanalyst would also limit contact with the psychopharmacologist as much as possible because doing so engages the analyst in nonanalytic interventions that impair analytic functioning. The analyst would not encourage or oppose the psychopharmacologist's interventions, but would explore the patient's reactions to the medication and the psychopharmacologist as they emerge in the therapy.

In our view, use of the abstinent model in this way impairs the psychoanalyst's ability to address medication appropriately with the psychopharmacologist. Clinically, many psychoanalysts feel that communication with the psychopharmacologist does not adversely affect their analytic function or is less likely to do so than prescribing the medication directly. As with any issue, therapists should be alert to the possibility that their view of the patient is being affected by a variety of factors, including feelings about the psychopharmacologist and medication, and be alert to disruptions in their therapeutic stance toward patients.

Communication After the Initial Consultation

In many instances, there is minimal communication after the psychopharmacologist initially evaluates the patient and begins medication. To some extent, this would be more in accord with Kelly's (1998) views described earlier. However, Gould and Busch (1998) suggest that there are certain key times when the therapist and psychopharmacologist should discuss the patient directly. These occasions include

> (1) when concerns about patients arise, (2) when significant treatment changes or recommendations for changes are made, (3) when one of the practitioners disagrees with the other's treatment, and (4) when the patient complains about one practitioner to the other. (p. 744)

For example, a psychopharmacologist was seeing a patient, Ms. SS, who had presented with depression and alcohol problems and responded well to sertraline 200 mg/day and behavioral changes with alcohol. The relationship among psychopharmacologist, therapist, and patient had been a positive one, and in general there had been little communication about the patient because she had improved with medication and had few problems with maintenance. After 1½ years on the medication, Ms. SS had been discussing tapering the medication with the psychiatrist and therapist, and at this particular session, the psychopharmacologist was to provide a tapering schedule. However, as the psychopharmacologist was assessing the patient, she revealed that her drinking had increased.

Psychopharmacologist: So how have things been going with your drinking?

Ms. SS: Not as well as it had been. There were a couple times when I felt I wasn't in such good control.

Psychopharmacologist: So what are your thoughts about tapering the medication, given that alcohol was an important precipitant of your depression?

Ms. SS: Well, I don't think it's a big deal. It's not really like I used to drink.

Psychopharmacologist: My concern is that your drinking has increased. Have you discussed this with your therapist?

Ms. SS: Yes. I told her about it, but she didn't seem terribly concerned.

Psychopharmacologist: I think it would be good for me to talk to her about the situation.

Ms. SS: Sure. I think it's a good idea.

The psychopharmacologist was concerned that the therapist was either unaware of or not adequately aggressive in addressing Ms. SS's substance abuse. Direct contact would help to clarify these issues:

Psychopharmacologist: I'm concerned that Ms. SS is not adequately acknowledging the problem with her drinking.

Therapist: Yes. I noticed the same thing. I've been attempting to address it with her. On the other hand, she does not want to feel controlled in the treatment, and I'm concerned that she may act out by rebelling and drinking more.

Psychopharmacologist: Have you discussed this concern with her?

Therapist: No. But it may be a good idea.

Psychopharmacologist: I think one way to address it more directly would be to state my concerns and the need to monitor alcohol more closely, especially when considering a reduction in medication. Perhaps that would take some of the heat off you.

Therapist: Okay. I'm going to talk to her about it.

At the next meeting with the psychopharmacologist Ms. SS revealed that she had reduced her drinking and was keeping a closer watch for it. They decided to proceed with the medication taper.

When communication does not occur in the instances described previously, problems can result. For example, Gould and Busch (1998) described a case in which a patient presented to the psychopharmacologist with a plan to taper off medication to pursue pregnancy. The psychopharmacologist viewed the decision as precipitous and recommended that the patient give further consideration to this issue before embarking on this plan. It later emerged that the patient had been discussing this with the therapist for some time and that the therapist recommended that she proceed. Tensions emerged that caused a temporary disruption in the triadic therapeutic alliance, but subsequent discussions between the clinicians helped to resolve this, including clarifying that major changes in treatment plans should be addressed directly between them.

Confidentiality

Communication between practitioners raises issues about confidentiality among therapist, psychopharmacologist, and patient. Generally, there should be an initial discussion with the patient clarifying that information can be shared between therapist and psychopharmacologist to prevent future misunderstandings. However, confidentiality concerns are sometimes not adequately discussed, and it is presumed that the patient understands that the clinicians will communicate. Unfortunately, this can lead to subsequent problems in the treatment. Two such instances are those in which a patient is upset that communication has taken place, or the patient requests that one of the practitioners not share information with the other.

If there has not been recent contact and practitioners plan to talk about a problem or disagreement, it is helpful to alert the patient, as was done in the treatment of Ms. SS described earlier. In the following case, communication between the therapist and a psychopharmacologist that was not mentioned ahead of time to the patient created distress for her.

Ms. TT, a 45-year-old single woman, had a depression that was initially responsive to a variety of medications, but kept recurring. The psychopharmacologist eventually discussed a possible trial of MAO inhibitors with the patient. In this context, he felt it would be important to alert the therapist to this possibility, given the issues that these medications would raise, such as dietary restrictions and possible health risks. He assumed that the patient would not have a problem with this communication because the therapist and psychopharmacologist had been in contact in the past, though not for some time. Unexpectedly, Ms. TT became angry that this discussion had taken place, feeling that the clinicians had gone behind her back. Exploration with the therapist was useful in understanding the origins of the patient's concerns (particularly, a mother who broadcast personal information about the patient to the mother's friends). While this led to productive therapeutic work, the psychopharmacologist agreed that alerting the patient about the contact would have been less disruptive.

Another issue arises when a patient asks the therapist or psychopharmacologist to withhold particular information from the other clinician. This request can represent several fantasies or conflicts. One motive may be to gain one clinician's collusion in devaluing the other. An example would be a patient who states to the psychopharmacologist that she is thinking about leaving her therapist because she feels the therapy is unproductive, but does not want the therapist to know. Encouraging the patient to address the problem directly to the clinician can be effective. The psychopharmacologist can explain to the patient that negative feelings about the therapist are important to talk about directly, both for the purpose of understanding them and to determine if the impasse can be resolved.

In some instances, however, the patient may be unwilling to express the concerns directly. In general, practitioners should avoid accepting the patient's request not to communicate. A useful approach is to discuss with the patient that asking the clinician not to reveal information puts him or her in a difficult position. First, it affects an agreement the practitioners had to communicate about problems, even if the patient is not recognizing this agreement. In addition, it interferes with the clinician helping the patient address the problem with the other practitioner. When the patient presents a concern about the psychopharmacologist, the problem can be more manageable because the therapist can dynamically explore the patient's concerns about revealing the problem. Sometimes such efforts represent a repeat of patterns in which a patient colluded with one parent regarding another, or it may indicate a fear of directly expressing negative feelings.

Another basis of a request not to share information is to avoid revealing something about which the patient is embarrassed. For instance, Ms. UU told her therapist that she did not want to discuss issues about plastic surgery with the male psychopharmacologist because "I don't need to talk to a man about my body." The therapist explored the threat the patient felt, in part related to a father who was intrusive regarding boundaries with her sexuality. The therapist contacted the psychopharmacologist, who clarified that while the patient need not go into detail, discussion of the surgery was important with regard to medication adjustments. The patient talked about the issue with the psychopharmacologist and later told the therapist that this experience was helpful, in that the psychopharmacologist was respectful of boundaries.

ISSUES OF RESPONSIBILITY

In cases where there are concerns about the patient's safety, responsibility for the patient's care usually falls to the psychopharmacologist. This is based on the psychopharmacologist's typically greater experience with cases in which there are safety concerns and the capacity to hospitalize a patient. There are, however, no absolute rules about how to handle these situations, and they are often subject to communication, consultation, and thoughtful discussion between the practitioners. Ultimately, if there is a disagreement about the need for hospitalization, a consultant may be required to aid in the decision.

In one case, a 26-year-old man in therapy was referred to a psychopharmacologist when he developed the onset of depressive symptoms with irritability in the context of struggles with work and a divorce. After feeling rejected by a friend, Mr. VV experienced suicidal ideation with thoughts of jumping from his window. The patient also described intermittent periods of feeling "up" with increased energy lasting a few days. The therapist was quite concerned about the patient's suicide risk, but the psychopharmacologist, on evaluating the patient, felt the risk was low. Mr. VV had reported some easing of depressive symptoms, stated they were due to very specific stressors, and denied current suicidal ideation. The psychopharmacologist made a diagnosis of bipolar, type II disorder, based on the history of the patient's symptoms and a family history of bipolar disorder, and recommended treatment with lamotrigene. The patient was resistant to this recommendation and wanted to meet with his therapist before starting it.

Approximately 4 days later, however, the patient had a bout of drinking after a conflict with his boss and reported spending 30 minutes looking over the edge of his balcony on the 12th floor, contemplating jumping. The therapist contacted the psychopharmacologist, expressing some frustration that he did not recognize the degree of suicidality and suggesting the patient may need to be hospitalized. The psychopharmacologist admitted that he needed to reevaluate his view, but the possibility of the patient having borderline personality features, with dramatic efforts to engage attention and unconsciously split the treatment team, also arose. Mr. VV agreed to start the medication before seeing the psychopharmacologist, but this medication would take some time to be adjusted to an adequate dose. In addition, the practitioners determined that the patient had to be warned about his drinking, which exacerbated his feelings of distress.

When the psychopharmacologist saw the patient the next day, he denied any further suicidal ideation since the incident 2 days previously. He accepted that drinking was a problem and was willing to discontinue it. Although he had agreed to start medication, he still struggled with the need for it. He felt that he had been dealing with mood fluctuations over many years, that these were more intense currently due to stressors, and that he wished to pursue a psychotherapeutic approach for now. The psychopharmacologist and therapist prevailed on him to continue his medication, particularly given his suicidality, and the psychopharmacologist prescribed risperidone, as needed, for when the patient was experiencing increased distress. Despite the episode of suicidality, he still did not find Mr. VV to be an acute suicide risk and felt that a hospitalization could be problematically disruptive for the patient. He again reassured the therapist, who continued to be quite concerned, but agreed to the plan.

Over the next few weeks the patient became calmer and less depressed, particularly in the context of further progress in his divorce, an easing of work stress, and decreased alcohol. Additionally, his therapist's reduced anxiety may have helped her to calm the patient. The patient discontinued the medication and was unwilling to restart, although he stated he would reconsider if his symptoms recurred or intensified. He showed no further signs of suicidality, and he terminated with the psychopharmacologist, with an agreement to return if there were subsequent symptoms.

MANAGEMENT OF A COMPLEX CASE

The following case describes a successful negotiation of a variety of potential conflicts with a borderline patient. The therapist and psychopharmacologist employed the principles of active communication about problems, avoidance of collusion, and maintenance of a triadic therapeutic alliance.

Ms. WW, a 21-year-old woman, presented to her therapist with depressive symptoms and described an intense struggle between her and her parents over her boyfriend, whom her parents ordered her to give up. The patient did not heed their demands and continued to see the boyfriend covertly. The therapist explored the patient's frustration about feeling controlled by her parents and the angry pressure she felt to rebel. With Ms. WW present, she met with the boyfriend and also felt concerned about whether he was appropriate for her, although she did not express this directly to the patient. She also sent the patient for psychopharmacology consultation. The psychopharmacologist evaluated the patient, felt her to have symptoms of a major depressive disorder, and recommended a trial of sertraline.

At this point the conflict between the patient and parents escalated. Ms. WW reported that her mother was frequently tearful, and woke the patient up repeatedly during the night to express her concerns. Both parents stated that the patient was "killing her mother." The parents went as far as to threaten payment of her college tuition if she kept in contact with the boyfriend. In addition, the parents were angry about the medication, expressing a wish that the patient discontinue it and accusing Ms. WW of manipulating the psychiatrist to prescribe in an attempt to get their sympathy. They threatened not to pay for the medication. The therapist, psychopharmacologist, and Ms. WW felt the parents should come in for a meeting with the therapist, but they initially refused. After a conflict that became physical, the patient moved out of the home to live with friends.

In this context the parents agreed to see the therapist. In addition to discussing the parents' concerns and the problematic effort to control Ms. WW, the therapist explained the value of medication for depressive symptoms. Reluctantly, the parents agreed to cover the costs, allowing Ms. WW to continue taking the sertraline, which had relieved her depressive symptoms. The therapist felt she was making progress with the parents, but 1 week later the therapist and psychopharmacologist received letters dismissing them from the case. The patient was contacted and was unaware of these letters and stated she would speak with the parents.

Two days later the psychopharmacologist received an urgent call from the parents, stating Ms. WW was "not herself." The patient, back at home with the parents, was labile, tearful, and disorganized. The psychopharmacologist agreed to a meeting with the parents and patient the next day and informed the therapist of the events. At this meeting the parents reported that Ms. WW had admitted using significant amounts of cocaine in the preceding 2 weeks, and the patient concurred with this. The parents noted that they were now aware that they had been too controlling and were backing off threats about college, allowing Ms. WW to see her boyfriend. However, they continued to express strong reservations about the medication. In addition, they questioned why the patient needed to see the therapist, and the patient stated that she "did not feel connected" with the therapist. The psychopharmacologist maintained a stance that Ms. WW should return to the therapist, especially because the therapist knew her better and could help sort out what steps to take. In addition, he recommended evaluation by a substance-abuse psychiatrist.

A few days later Ms. WW did see the therapist. Her mood was labile, and she seemed "high." It was unclear whether she was demonstrating signs of a bipolar, type II disorder, affective lability as part of a borderline personality disorder, or the effects of cocaine. She contacted the psychopharmacologist, and after evaluating the patient, he decreased the sertraline dosage to 100 mg/day. The next day, the patient took an overdose of clonazepam. After 2 days in the hospital, she was found not to be a suicide risk and was discharged.

At this point, efforts shifted to finding a substance-abuse program for the patient, as well as ongoing work with the patient and parents. Ms. WW's condition improved markedly as she avoided cocaine and alcohol. Despite their stated intent, the parents continued to attempt to control her treatment. They wanted the patient to change psychiatrists and refused substance-abuse consultation. They were preoccupied with the patient's social activities, attempting to prevent her from any contacts with others who might be using drugs. Ms. WW expressed desperation, annoyance, and sometimes rage at the parents. Indeed, the therapist and psychopharmacologist admitted to each other that they occasionally struggled with similar feelings toward the parents. In this way they were able to discuss pressures they felt from the parents to change treatment according to their wishes and empathy for the position of the patient. They pressed the parents to enter into therapy focused on their parenting issues. These ongoing efforts helped to ease Ms. WW's distress regarding her parents.

This enormously complex case demonstrates how combined treatment may work well with a psychopharmacologist and psychotherapist involved in the case. Efforts to split the treatment team by both the parents and the patient were unsuccessful due to communication and support between the practitioners. It was the awareness of these potential problems that allowed the therapist and psychopharmacologist to recognize these behaviors and attitudes and to address them appropriately. In addition, efforts were made to engage the patient in a triadic therapeutic alliance that helped her to resist her parents' efforts to split and undermine the treatment, helping her become a more active participant in her own care.

8

Combined Treatment for Depressive and Anxiety Disorders

With the exception of personality disorders (discussed in chapter 5), therapists working with patients in combined treatment will primarily be addressing depressive and anxiety disorders. These diagnoses are common in this population, and many of the examples presented thus far have involved patients with these diagnoses. This chapter is designed to discuss the particular dynamics and special issues that emerge in psychotherapeutic and pharmacological interventions in these cases.

COMBINED TREATMENT OF DEPRESSION

As discussed in chapter 2, patients often have both psychological and chemical vulnerabilities to depressive disorders. One metaphor for understanding these contributions, described earlier, is that of tributaries (chemical, psychological, environmental) to a river, where overflow is equivalent to a depressive disorder. In addition, chemical and psychological vulnerabilities can interact. For example, chemical factors contribute to low self-esteem, which can trigger dynamic factors that intensify depressive symptoms (such as the vicious cycles described later). As noted in chapter 5, medication can help to "clear up the field" by treating chemical factors and assessing what symptoms persist.

Evidence continues to grow that combined treatment can have advantages over psychotherapy or medication alone. For example, a large multicenter study on the combined treatment of chronic major depression compared a form of cognitive behavioral treatment—cognitive behavioral analysis system of psychotherapy (CBASP)—with the antidepressant nefazodone and a combination of the two treatments (Keller et al., 2000). The treatments lasted for 12 weeks with patients who had been ill for at least 2 years. The study showed a significant advantage of combined treatment over either monotherapy.

Controversy continues in terms of whether depressive symptoms or traits not at the level of a major depressive disorder always represent dysthymic disorder or could also be character elements of a depressive personality disorder. In making a distinction, proponents of depressive personality disorder describe its criteria as primarily psychological, as opposed to the primarily somatic and vegetative symptoms of dysthymia (McDermut, Zimmerman, & Chelminski, 2003; Ryder, Bagby, & Schuller, 2002). In depressive personality disorder, mood disturbance need not be central to the diagnosis, and the diagnosis is conceptualized as persisting traits rather than symptoms, particularly "excessive negative, pessimistic beliefs about oneself and other people" (Hirschfeld & Holzer, 1994).

In a study of adult psychiatric outpatients, McDermut et al. (2003) found that depressive personality disorder was not redundant with other Axis I or II disorders. Depressive personality disorder was associated with greater comorbidity (particularly anxiety disorders), more impaired psychosocial functioning, and higher rates of mood disorders and alcohol abuse in relatives, compared to psychiatric patients without depressive personality disorder. Alternatively, Ryder et al. (2002) argue that "despite persuasive evidence for the existence of depressive personality traits, support is insufficient for the inclusion of depressive personality disorder as currently defined" (p. 337). No medication studies have been done on depressive personality disorder to assess if symptoms respond. Therapists, however, need to be alert to the possibility that persistent depressive symptoms may represent ongoing chemical vulnerabilities that could be further diminished with additional medication intervention.

For instance, Ms. XX had a high chronic expectation of rejection from others. She felt that, unless she was warmly regarded by everyone she knew, that meant she was being rejected. In fact, Ms. XX simply felt as if rejection were taking place and would search out some kind of evidence to confirm that it was occurring. Psychiatric evaluation indicated the presence of a major depressive disorder, with a panoply of cognitive and vegetative symptoms. In addition, Ms. XX's developmental history suggested a variety of psychological vulnerabilities, based on a family background that included an intensely critical mother and a neglectful father focused on his business activities. In essence, Ms. XX felt rejected by her parents, and her subsequent expectations of rejection appeared to mirror this pattern.

After treatment with an antidepressant (she responded well to higher doses of venlafaxine), Ms. XX's depressive and vegetative symptoms eased significantly, but her expectation of rejection continued to be very strong. The psychiatrist/therapist viewed these remaining symptoms as depressive personality traits and therefore shifted to a predominantly psychotherapeutic approach. He helped Ms. XX to understand her expectation of rejection as related to early traumatic experiences, and he looked at how her angry reactions to these expectations became internalized, leading to intense self-criticism.

Despite an increasingly sophisticated conception of the dynamics by therapist and patient, the intensity of Ms. XX's low self-esteem persisted. The therapist wondered whether anything more might be done to ease these symptoms with additional pharmacological intervention, despite the absence of vegetative symptoms. In terms presented previously, the therapist was assessing whether the patient had an obstruction (an ongoing chemical vulnerability), rather than a resistance, to psychotherapy. He decided to recommend the addition of bupropion, to which the patient agreed. This intervention led to a further reduction in her expectation of rejection and feelings of inadequacy, which aided the therapist and patient in insight-oriented work. The case suggests the need for ongoing attention to both chemical and psychological contributors to symptoms in the treatment of depression.

Dynamics of Depression

Psychoanalysts have been writing about the dynamics of depression since early in the development of psychoanalytic theory and clinical work. Awareness of these dynamic factors can guide therapists in their psychodynamic psychotherapeutic interventions and are also relevant to medication management in a combined treatment. Drawing from the work of several psychoanalytic theorists and research on psychological factors in depression, Busch, Rudden, and Shapiro (2004) delineated five central dynamics in depressive disorders. These include:

- Narcissistic vulnerability: This refers to a sensitivity to perceived or actual losses or rejections. Individuals with narcissistic vulnerability will tend to perceive more events as rejections or losses and react to them with a greater degree of loss of self-esteem, depressive affects, and rage.
- Conflicted anger: Anger at others is experienced as either difficult to tolerate or unacceptable, triggering self-criticism and/or guilt. These reactions can indicate a turning of anger against the self.
- Severe superego: The superego represents the conscience function of the individual; patients who are vulnerable to depression are likely to have a particularly harsh or rigid superego. The severe superego is associated with an intolerance of a variety of feelings, including anger, sexuality, and envy, leading to self-criticisms, an associated lowering of self-esteem, and expectations of punishment.

- Idealized and devalued perceptions of self and others: Patients prone to depression will tend to idealize others with a fantasy that connections with them will compensate for their low self-esteem. However, these idealizations often lead to disappointment and depression. Patients may devalue others to bolster their own self-esteem and to protect against feeling rejected.
- Defense mechanisms: To protect themselves from painful affects, depressed patients tend to employ particular defenses, such as denial, projection, passive aggression, and reaction formation. However, these defenses paradoxically exacerbate depression, as patients are not able to deal directly with the feelings that are being triggered. For instance, anger that is projected leads to experiencing others as more negative or critical, passive aggression tends to arouse ire in others, and reaction formation can lead to individuals being overly nice to those with whom they are angry.

Cognition, affects, and conflicts involved in the dynamics of depression lead to vicious cycles that intensify depressive affects. In one formulation, perceived rejection triggers anger as described previously. This anger, which causes conflict, shifts to guilt and self-criticism. The self-criticism intensifies feelings of low self-esteem, which increases the sense of rejection and level of narcissistic vulnerability.

In a second vicious cycle, low self-esteem leads to a propensity to idealize others to ease low self-esteem. However, this idealization often triggers disappointment and devaluation of self and others, with a further lowering of self-esteem.

Depressive Dynamics and Combined Treatment

The dynamics of depression described earlier affect patients' expectations of and reactions to medication. The experience of shame in response to medication was discussed in chapter 5, in a case that focused on fears of lack of control of feelings, related to identification with the mother (Ms. EE). If patients have a sensitivity to rejection or perceive experiences in the context of their low self-esteem, the recommendation of medication can be viewed as another narcissistic injury.

For example, Busch et al. (2004) described the case of a patient (Ms. AAA) who saw the need for medication as a sign of being defective in some way. Associated with this feeling of being flawed was a sense that others would reject her for taking medication. This reflected her self-view—particularly as an adolescent, when she felt ignored by her father and by her classmates, viewing herself as unappealing and unattractive. These feelings led the patient repeatedly to reduce the dose of her medication, leading to exacerbation of her depression, a furthering decrease in self-esteem, and additional humiliation triggered by evidence of her need for medication. Exploration of the link of medication to experiences of feeling ignored or rejected in adolescence improved her attitude about medication and increased her compliance.

Difficulties With Anger Management

Patients with depression often struggle with angry reactions toward others, often resulting from feelings of narcissistic injury. This anger is usually experienced as threatening, so it will often emerge indirectly. For instance, anger can be denied and take the form of passive aggression, projection, or reaction formation, defenses found in depression as noted before. The following case describes an instance where passive aggression became involved in the medication treatment, allowing exploration of this issue and a link to other instances where this defense was operative.

Ms. YY, a 45-year-old woman with a long history of recurrent severe depression, had a fear of expressing her anger that stemmed from several sources. She was concerned that others would reject her if she became angry. In addition, she was worried about being hurtful or damaging to others through expression of her anger. Each of these fears mirrored her experience of her mother, who withdrew from the patient in silence for days if one of the children got mad at her, and viciously attacked others in a way that disrupted her close relationships.

Because of her intolerance of anger, Ms. YY would often behave in a highly passive–aggressive manner, resisting the expectations others had of her. For instance, Ms. YY would come late to work, even when she knew that her boss was particularly troubled by this behavior. The therapist would interpret the patient's underlying anger, which she typically denied; she stated that the problem stemmed from difficulties with the snooze button on her alarm. However, over time the therapist was able to point out a pattern in which Ms. YY's passive–aggressive behavior would follow episodes in which the boss behaved in ways she found hurtful.

At one point, Ms. YY became frustrated about a planned reduction in frequency of visits from twice to once a week, even though she had agreed to this plan based on her improvement and wish to save money. In this context, there was a temporary worsening of her depression. As the therapist was exploring the sources of her depression, including feelings of loss of the therapist, Ms. YY revealed that she had been "forgetting" doses of medication. Ms. YY denied being angry at the therapist and did not connect this with her forgetting medication. As this pattern continued, the therapist worked to link this pattern to Ms. YY's anger.

Therapist: What happens when you forget your medication?

Ms. YY: I'm not sure. I mean to take it, but I usually take it at work because I don't have time in the morning, and then work gets too busy.

Therapist: But this did not happen before we planned to reduce the frequency of your sessions.

Ms. YY: No. Only occasionally. I know you see the two events as connected, but I really don't feel that.

Therapist: Well, it seems similar to your behavior with your boss. When he criticizes you, you'll often oversleep and come late to work. We've found that somehow when you're angry you don't realize it and you express it in this indirect way.

Ms. YY: It does seem similar to that pattern.

Therapist: How are you feeling about the reduction in visits?

Ms. YY: Well, it's been difficult. I miss coming here. And sometimes I wish you could reduce your fee to make it easier for me.

Therapist: Well, perhaps you're angry at me about that.

Ms. YY: Yes. I guess that's possible.

Guilt and the Severe Superego

As noted before, patients with depression often struggle with the sense that they have done something wrong and should be punished in some way for this. Often these fantasies relate to conflicts about particular kinds of feelings, including angry, vengeful, dependent, or sexual feelings that are felt to be intolerable or unacceptable. In psychoanalytic terms, this is conceptualized as a severe superego—the conscience function that monitors the individual's thoughts, feelings, and behaviors, rendering some form of judgment as to whether they are acceptable, and determining whether praise or punishment should be meted out. Although not a focus in the case involving a negative reaction to effective medication described in chapter 5, the severe superego can affect the tolerance of positive results from medication. Patients may feel they do not deserve the improvement they are getting, or may be threatened by the potential to experience more actively the intense feelings that trigger guilt.

Ms. ZZ, for example, was a 35-year-old woman with a history of recurrent depression. Contributing to her depression was the tendency toward reaction formation, often doing things for others even if she was angry with them. For instance, Ms. ZZ regularly arranged visits with her father at his request, even though he often canceled them or ridiculed her when they got together. He was critical about a variety of her behaviors: her clothing, work, and friends. If she did not get together with him, she felt guilty, with a sense that she was hurting him and he would feel sad and lonely. In therapy, Ms. ZZ also became aware of a fantasy that if she were nice to her father at some point he would suddenly become nice to her. Therefore, she hesitated to confront him about his attitudes. However, she was recurrently disappointed after these efforts did not lead to positive changes in their relationship.

As she improved with antidepressants, Ms. ZZ began to shift in her attitudes toward her father. At that time her father had setbacks in his work and with a woman to whom he was engaged. Ms. ZZ noticed herself having the thought, "Now he can see what it's like to suffer. I hope he loses his job and his girlfriend." Whereas in the past intense guilt would have precluded any conscious awareness of vengeful fantasies, she was now able to talk to her therapist about these feelings. However, direct expression of the fantasy triggered a wave of guilt.

Ms. ZZ: I don't think it's right to have this kind of thought.
Therapist: What do you feel is the problem with it?
Ms. ZZ: It's mean. I don't really want him to suffer. Do other people have these kinds of thoughts?
Therapist: They're actually quite common. We need to understand what upsets you so much about it. It doesn't seem as if you're actually acting in a vengeful way toward your father.
Ms. ZZ: I felt certain you were going to be critical of my thinking this—that you wouldn't want to be with me.
Therapist: It sounds like the kind of criticism you often expect from your father.
Ms. ZZ: Yes. That's true. And, no, I haven't been mean to him. In fact, I'm still too nice!

The therapist's nonjudgmental stance furthered Ms. ZZ's ability to tolerate and explore fantasies of revenge. Work with both medication and therapy eased the restrictions of her superego, the guilt she experienced, and the punishment she thought she deserved. As she became more comfortable with criticisms of her father, the reaction formation diminished, and she was able to set better limits and become more tolerant of not being able to develop a closer relationship with him.

Idealization and Devaluation

Partly related to current cultural factors in the United States (see chapter 4), patients can develop very high expectations of what medication can accomplish for them. One basis for this expectation is direct-to-consumer advertising, which paints a very positive portrait of medication. It is not unusual for patients presenting with a request for a medication seen on a commercial. In addition, *Listening to Prozac* (Kramer, 1993) was interpreted by many readers as an indicator that problems previously viewed as personality difficulties could respond to medication interventions; patients would allude to examples in the book of people who felt "better than ever" on Prozac.

Per the dynamics discussed previously, medication may be idealized in an attempt to relieve depression and low self-esteem. However, this idealization greatly increases the propensity to disappointment and, subsequently, devaluation, which can worsen depression and further disrupt therapy. The next case describes a patient whose tendency to idealize and devalue affected her experience of medication.

Ms. AAA was a 32-year-old woman with a long history of depression who presented with typical symptoms of a major depressive episode. She reported that she had felt the best she ever had, "better than normal," for a brief period when she first went on fluoxetine 5 years previously. Although it was possible that Ms. AAA had a hypomanic response to medication, she denied other signs and symptoms of hypomania. However, after about a month, her "usual" mood returned. Since then she had undergone numerous medication trials, but the intense positive feeling had never returned. Ms. AAA stated that she had come in specifically to find a medication that made her feel the same way.

Ms. AAA described a series of disrupted relationships with men that were reminiscent psychologically of her experience with medication. She developed intensely positive feelings for them and was subsequently disappointed by their behavior, after which she broke up with them. Although this pattern suggested a co-occurring diagnosis of narcissistic personality disorder, Ms. AAA was not interested in psychotherapy for these problems. She stated that if she found the right medication, she would feel better, and she hoped the doctor would provide that. In a similar fashion to her other patterns, she had heard very positive things about the psychiatrist's psychopharmacological skills and hoped he could find the needed medication.

The therapist responded that he would certainly try to find an effective medication (there were a few medications that had not been tried), but he was concerned that the desired effect would not be achieved and that she would be disappointed in him as well. He also suggested psychotherapy to better understand her pattern of intense excitement about relationships and the first medication, followed by severe disappointment. However, Ms. AAA maintained that she was not interested in psychotherapy. After two medication trials that did not achieve the desired result, she dropped out of treatment.

In addition to the pattern of idealization, Ms. AAA also devalued the therapist, not accepting his suggestions on what might be helpful. Devaluation can reflect a self-critical feeling arising out of guilt and/or a projection onto others of feelings of worthlessness. In addition, a patient can devalue others in order to boost his self-esteem. Unfortunately, this negative view reduces the value of others in the patient's mind, diminishing the potential to feel helped or supported by others. In addition, as noted earlier, devaluation can increase the pressure toward idealization to relieve depression, creating a vicious cycle. This cycle may have been involved in Ms. AAA's patterns with the psychiatrists and medication.

In a related vein, patients may devalue medications before actually receiving them. Patients may state that medication will be ineffective, due to the severity of their depression or by seeing others, including the psychopharmacologist, as unable to help them. Additionally, patients may claim that the medication would be damaging to them because these agents are not "natural."

Countertransference With Depressed Patients

Several countertransference problems can affect the combined treatment of depressed patients. Particularly in more severe cases, therapists can develop countertransference feelings that match the patient's pessimism and experience feelings of hopelessness and inadequacy about their treatment. This negative view can occur in response to patients' efforts, both conscious and unconscious, to convince therapists that their situations are hopeless. The development of this attitude is more likely if patients are dealing with setbacks in their lives, such as loss of a job, financial status, or important relationships. It is important to remember that patients can suffer from a depression no matter what their external circumstances are. Therapists need to be alert to a "giving up" that can cause less aggressive pharmacotherapeutic interventions or a feeling of impotence with psychotherapy.

For example, Mr. BBB suffered an exacerbation of a chronic depression after separation from his wife and loss of his job. He began to experience catastrophic feelings about his situation that were intensified by difficulty finding a new job. Mr. BBB presented an extended series of reasons as to why finding a job would be difficult, including his age and skill level. He was intensely self-critical about having been laid off, even though he had believed it would be good to leave and was finding the job intolerable.

The therapist found himself feeling increasingly concerned about the precariousness of Mr. BBB's situation. At that point, he recalled that Mr. BBB was similarly depressed when he was working and married. The patient had felt that he was consumed by the needs of others and could not follow his own interests. Leaving these situations had initially triggered a feeling of freedom that he had not experienced in many years.

Therapist: In our prior discussions you felt very upset by your marriage and your job.

Mr. BBB: Yes. That's true. But I hadn't anticipated the loneliness I would feel. And it's very strange not working. I had looked forward to going to museums, but there are only so many museums you can go to.

Therapist: I also think it's hard for you to adapt to the feeling of not having so many responsibilities. You've always felt under so much pressure to take care of others.

Mr. BBB: Yes. I felt very burdened by that. But I think it also helped me to feel important.

As the therapist recognized Mr. BBB's pessimism and self-criticism, he realized that the patient might be having a recurrence of depression. The therapist had been affected by Mr. BBB's presentation of negatives in his life, and this initially prevented his considering the possibility that the depression had returned. An evaluation revealed the presence of typical symptoms of a major depression. Therapist and patient then shifted to a discussion of an adjustment of Mr. BBB's medication, and it was determined that lamotrigine should be added to his current regimen. This intervention significantly relieved Mr. BBB's depression and helped him to pursue new job options and relationships. An exploration of his overresponsibility and caretaking of others was an important issue in the psychotherapy at this time.

Another countertransference response to depression occurs when patients present themselves as worthless and describe accepting mistreatment by others in their lives. Therapists may be affected by the sense that these patients do not deserve the usual care. In these instances, therapists should be alert to a propensity to reschedule patients frequently, not call in prescriptions quickly, or minimize side effects. An instance where this occurred is the case of Ms. Y, described in chapter 5, who accepted mistreatment by others in her life. After several instances in which the therapist requested a time change, she revealed that she felt as if the therapist viewed her as a second-class citizen. The therapist admitted his error in the frequent rescheduling, and they were able to explore this productively in psychotherapy.

Therapists also should be alert to anger in response to patients' resistance to medication, whether expressed indirectly through passive aggression, as in the earlier case of Ms. YY, or directly in rebellion, as noted in the case of Mr. DD in chapter 5. Additionally, therapists can get angry when patients do not improve, experiencing the stasis as a narcissistic injury to their therapeutic skills. Finally, in instances involving projection, therapists can be frustrated by patients' views of them as hurtful and rejecting.

Psychopharmacologists who are not as familiar with monitoring countertransference may be provoked by these various attitudes and behaviors into acting in rejecting ways, such as firing the patient. Nevertheless, even experienced therapists can be negatively affected by more complex depressed patients and need to be alert to more subtle manifestations of rejection. Thus, acknowledgment of countertransference is important to avert disruptions in psychotherapeutic and psychopharmacological care.

COMBINED TREATMENT OF ANXIETY DISORDERS

The focus of this section will be on panic disorder and generalized anxiety disorder (GAD), but aspects of the psychopharmacological and psychological theory and treatment of panic and GAD overlap with other anxiety disorders. In addition, we will briefly address issues in combined treatment of obsessive–compulsive disorder.

As with depressive disorders, anxiety disorders also likely derive from both chemical and psychological sources. Gorman, Kent, Sullivan, and Coplan (2000), for example, suggested that panic disorder involves an oversensitive fear network, comprising the prefrontal cortex, thalamus, amygdala, brainstem, hypothalamus, and other brain structures. The central component of this fear system is the amygdala, which coordinates physiological and behavioral reactions to danger. Both brainstem structures and cortical areas have input to the amygdala, allowing, respectively, an immediate and more processed response to danger. Relief of anxiety disorders from an oversensitive system can occur "top down," from psychotherapy increasing the ability of the cortical system to override automatic responses from the amygdala (Gorman et al., 2000; LeDoux, 1996), or "bottom up" through effecting an impact on brainstem and amygdala systems with medication.

Thus, the use of combined psychotherapy and medication is frequent in the treatment of these problems. Pharmacological treatment of anxiety disorders typically involves rapidly acting, as needed, use of benzodiazepine agents and/or longer term interventions with antidepressants with antianxiety functions that take effect gradually. The use of benzodiazepines can often allow patients to achieve a level of comfort while the therapist initiates psychotherapeutic management of the anxiety disorder, sometimes avoiding the need for an antidepressant. However, in instances of a more severe or persistent disorder, therapists often start antidepressants, but continue to work with a simultaneous psychotherapeutic intervention. Because medication efficacy has been demonstrated and some doctors and patients prefer it, many anxiety disorder patients are treated with medication alone.

As discussed later, anxiety disorders can relate psychologically to conflicts over angry and dependent feelings. Medication intervention may work to ease these conflicts by diminishing the vulnerability to irritability as well as anxiety, reducing the threat from angry and dependent wishes and impulses. In working with patients, a helpful metaphor describes anxiety as an overactivated alarm system that is triggered too easily or sounds a much louder alarm than is necessary. Medication and psychotherapy can each help to ease the catastrophic danger associated with anxiety disorders, calibrating the alarm system.

Notably, medication treatment of anxiety has been seen and is still viewed by some psychotherapists as disruptive of an exploratory psychodynamic process. In this conception, anxiety is of value as a motivator of treatment and as a signal of unconscious conflicts (see chapter 1); the signal suggests a pathway for the therapist and patient to explore to gain information about the patient's intrapsychic conflicts (Roose, 1995). One way to conceptualize this issue is that a certain level of anxiety is of value in this regard, but catastrophic levels of anxiety are disruptive rather than helpful. It is the catastrophic levels that are the intended target of medication. In some instances, patients will lose motivation for psychotherapy when their anxiety is relieved with medication. Depending on the particular circumstances, this may or may not be a problem with regard to therapeutic outcome.

Dynamics of Anxiety Disorders

From the psychodynamic perspective, anxiety disorders are typically viewed as related to unconscious or preconscious affects and wishes that are felt to be unsafe in some way or that trigger conflict. Prominent among these are angry feelings and fantasies, alongside dependency longings and wishes. Patients with anxiety disorders often experience insecure attachments and see their dependency wishes as dangerous because they feel they cannot safely count on others to respond to their needs and fears. In this context, vengeful feelings and fantasies can become particularly frightening as concerns emerge that the enactment of these wishes will cause a further disruption of the relationship with needed others.

These dynamics combine with different defense mechanisms and chemical vulnerabilities to produce the various anxiety disorders. In specific phobias, for example, anger is projected and displaced to objects in the environment, which are then avoided to ease the fear. In Freud's case of the child Little Hans (Freud, 1909a), the child's unconscious angry and competitive wishes toward his father were experienced as threatening. These wishes were then projected, seen as coming from the environment, and displaced onto horses, which symbolized the father. Thus, the patient feared that the horse (father) would damage him rather than that he would hurt his father.

In a psychodynamic investigation of panic disorder, Busch et al. (1991) and Shear et al. (1993) presented a model in which individuals prone to panic disorder develop a fearful dependency on others based on a neurophysiological vulnerability or traumatic developmental experiences. This fearful dependency, the sense that they are not safe without the presence of others, becomes a source of narcissistic humiliation as the individual feels incapable of managing independently. The humiliation leads to anger, but this anger creates anxiety because the individual fears damaging the relationship with the needed other.

Ultimately, a vicious cycle of fearful dependency, narcissistic humiliation, anger, increased anxiety, and fearful dependency occurs. Defenses are triggered, including reaction formation, undoing, and denial, that attempt to minimize anger and intensify affiliative efforts. However, these defenses prove unsuccessful, and the failure of the signal anxiety function of the ego leads to panic. Panic symptoms minimize access to anger and maintain attachment through a desperate plea for help.

Milrod, Busch, Cooper, and Shapiro (1997) identified four dynamic factors they found to be relevant to the psychopharmacological treatment of panic disorder; these overlap with issues found in anxiety disorders in general:

- Intense anxiety can be experienced as a sign of weakness, and patients often feel humiliated about the presence of severe anxiety. They may react by developing a counterphobic view of themselves as "strong." Thus, patients may view medication as a symbol of their weakness or struggle against medication because of the need to avoid feelings of humiliation.
- Recommendations for medication can arouse dependency wishes and conflicts in patients. They struggle between wishes to be cared for and fears they will be abandoned or intruded upon in response to dependency longings.
- Patients with anxiety disorders often have fears of losing control. These fears can be greatly intensified by medication and exacerbated by side effects. Fears of loss of control over their bodies can relate to frightening angry fantasies. These patients often need significant reassurance about the safety and value of medication.
- Fears and wishes regarding pregnancy as well as pregnancy itself constitute a special category of medication issues. Fears about pregnancy include fantasies of bodily damage and losing control, including concerns about harming the child. Additionally, becoming a mother often disrupts dependency wishes because of having to take care of others rather than be taken care of. Patients may avoid stopping medication as a rationalization to avoid pregnancy or have exacerbated concerns about bodily damage to themselves or the fetus from medication.

In addition to the dynamics described previously, anxiety symptoms both symbolize and avert frightening unconscious feelings and fantasies. Diminished anxiety symptoms with medication can bring these feelings more directly into consciousness. Improvement can also threaten dependency because the patient's symptomatic preoccupation may have been employed unconsciously to engender caretaking behavior from others. For these reasons, medication intervention can be experienced as threatening or destabilizing.

Feelings of Weakness and Needing Medication. As noted earlier, patients with anxiety disorders struggle with feelings of narcissistic injury about anxiety symptoms. Therefore they will sometimes find the need for medication to be humiliating. In addition, due to their internal representations of others as being rejecting or abandoning, anxious patients may anticipate the therapist behaving toward them in critical or humiliating ways. Anger that is denied can be projected onto others, exacerbating patients' experience that the therapist will be undermining or attacking. Thus, the introduction of medication could be interpreted in a similar way (e.g., the therapist pointing out that they are unable to function). Medication may also be viewed as suggesting that patients' fears are even less manageable than they have felt. Counterphobic efforts to be "strong," as a means of avoiding or denying anxiety and humiliation, can lead to struggles about the need for medication..

Ms. CCC, a 70-year-old woman, developed the onset of panic attacks associated with fears of being alone. She attributed her panic to breathing difficulties she associated with mild chronic obstructive pulmonary disease. However, her internist and pulmonologist felt that her medical condition could not account for the degree of difficulty that she experienced with her breathing. She presented on alprazolam 0.25 mg once a day, which she had been given by a psychiatrist in an emergency room, who had explained to her that she was having panic attacks. She also had developed depressed mood and mild vegetative symptoms, which she felt were secondary to her frustration with her anxiety. During the evaluation, Ms. CCC initially denied any preexisting anxiety or significant stressors.

The therapist suggested psychotherapy plus an increase in alprazolam to 0.25 to 0.5 mg every 4 to 6 hours as needed. Because of the severity of the panic and increasing depression, the therapist also suggested a trial of sertraline. Ms. CCC, however, was resistant to these suggestions, stating that she did not like taking medications. Over the next few days, Ms. CCC's panic persisted. In phone contacts, it emerged that Ms. CCC had not increased her alprazolam dose beyond the 0.25 mg daily dose she had started with, despite ongoing therapist suggestions. In addition, Ms. CCC was resistant to come in for additional sessions, stating she wished to go back to her country home.

In the next session, Ms. CCC discussed more about the history of her anxiety. She revealed that a milder form of anxiety had begun the previous summer. This was just after she was laid off her job as an editor, which she had had for over 40 years. She was both humiliated and angry that this had occurred, especially after her many years of service. She began to face the prospect of what she would do with more time and less structure in her life. Fortunately, work on her house commanded her attention, although she was more concerned about being able to pay for the work without her job.

Although in the city she had regular activities, when she had returned to her country home 2 months previously, she had felt there was too much time on her hands. While she had previously prided herself on her independence, she began to greatly miss her husband, who would come out only on weekends. At this point, she had the onset of panic and terror of being alone. Ms. CCC was humiliated by these symptoms, thus adding to her resistance to treatment, but felt desperate for help. The therapist explored these feelings in the context of medication treatment.

Therapist: You seem to be in a lot of conflict about getting help for this problem.

Ms. CCC: I hadn't really thought of it that way.

Therapist: Well, you want to come to sessions but then talk about leaving for the country as soon as possible, and you are reluctant to increase the medication to a higher dose.

Ms. CCC: I really don't like medication.

Therapist: What is it that you don't like about it?

Ms. CCC: I'm not really sure.

Therapist: From what you told me I wonder if you feel embarrassed about needing it—that it's a sign of how much help you need when you're used to being so independent.

Ms. CCC: Well, that could be true. I certainly don't like being in this position.

Conflicts About Dependency and Taking Medication As described earlier, patients with anxiety often suffer from dependency conflicts that stem from and exacerbate their anxiety. Patients long for caring from others, but also struggle with these wishes. Sources of these conflicts include humiliation about needing help and fears that others will respond to their needs with abandonment or intrusion. However, the effort to deny dependency wishes often only exacerbates them because patients become unable to communicate directly about the response they desire from others. As noted previously, these conflicts can involve medication: Patients long for the relief it may provide, but fear the dependency that the medication signifies.

For example, dependency conflicts played a role in Ms. CCC's struggle with medication. Curiously, fears of becoming dependent were focused on antidepressants rather than benzodiazepines, which do contain some risks of physiological dependency. These concerns in part related to her feelings of humiliation in needing medication as described before. There was a long-standing focus on viewing herself as independent, capable of handling things on her own emotionally. This appeared to derive in part from problems in her early life resulting from a mostly absent alcoholic father, and a frequently absent mother who had to work two jobs in order to support the family. The need to manage on her own was linked to an identification with her mother and a counterphobic need to deny her intense longing for care, which had been met in very limited ways. Thus, Ms. CCC found benzodiazepines, where she made the decision to take them, less threatening than antidepressants, which she perceived as being imposed on her.

Ms. CCC: I don't want to be dependent on the medication.
Therapist: What do you mean by that?
Ms. CCC: You know. End up having to take it for the rest of your life.
Therapist: Actually, antidepressants really don't have a risk of dependency in the way that people usually think of it. It's not that if you stop you would feel a pressure or urge to take the medication.
Ms. CCC: Well, that may be, but I still don't like it.
Therapist: I wonder if part of the issue is that for so long you've been doing things independently. From what you told me you've felt on your own much of the time since you were a child. It's important for you, but it's been much harder since you've lost your job, since you have to lean on others.
Ms. CCC: My mother didn't like us to bother her much. She was very busy just trying to keep the household going. And I don't think my husband likes it either. He's not used to my being like this. He gets really annoyed.
Therapist: Well, I think these are important issues to work out, but I think that the medication has become caught up in your conflicts and fears about being taken care of. You feel that, if you are not deciding when to take the medication or feel dependent on it, you may end up feeling rejected.
Ms. CCC: Well, I'm certainly not used to being in this position, and I guess the medication reminds me of needing help.

Ongoing explorations of Ms. CCC's feelings of humiliation and fears of dependency were of value both in her increasing acceptance of medication and in understanding how these conflicts affected her anxiety more generally.

Fears of Loss of Control Fear of losing control is a central feature of the dynamics of anxiety disorders. Patients typically fear, usually unconsciously, the emergence of forbidden feelings and fantasies. They are concerned these dependent and angry wishes will be expressed in ways that are damaging to themselves and others. Medication will often become caught in these conflicts because patients' fears can be projected onto the medication, which then becomes a source or expression of fantasies of damaging loss of control.

Ms. DDD was a 43-year-old mother of two whose panic attacks emerged in the context of fights with her older child, a daughter who was 15 years old. Ms. DDD was aware of being "too nice" with her daughter and had trouble setting limits. She quickly grasped that this was part of a more general pattern of unassertiveness. This included fears of confronting a temperamental and alcoholic father, a frequently absent mother, and a controlling, domineering older sister. Unconsciously utilizing reaction formation, Ms. DDD became "too nice" to others with the hope that her attachments would be less disrupted and she would not drive others away.

Because of the severity of her panic attacks and some mild depressive symptoms, the therapist/psychiatrist decided to begin a sertraline trial. Recognizing the importance of beginning medication at low doses in patients with anxiety, Ms. DDD started on 25 mg/day. However, on this dose, her reaction was quite severe: She experienced palpitations, intense anxiety, and feelings of being out of control shortly after taking her first pill. It was difficult to differentiate her usual panic from the reaction to medication that she described; however, Ms. DDD was convinced medication was the culprit. She agreed to take 12.5 mg/day, but had a similar reaction. The therapist addressed Ms. DDD's reaction with her.

Ms. DDD: I don't want to try it again. I'm afraid of losing control.
Therapist: This is a very strong reaction to this low dose of medication. I'm not sure what you mean when you say you're afraid of losing control.
Ms. DDD: I'm not sure either. But I was thinking about it and I do know that my father and sister have terrible tempers. I know that my father was out of control when he was angry.
Therapist: So you feel you might be worried about losing control of your anger?
Ms. DDD: I guess so.
Therapist: Are you angry about taking the medication?
Ms. DDD: I'm not sure. I know you want me to take it, but I'm not sure if I want to.
Therapist: Well, I guess we need to discuss this further, as these feelings seem to be increasing your anxiety right now. It seems like you are being "nice" with me like you often are with others.
Ms. DDD: Possibly.

Further psychotherapeutic work in Ms. DDD's case confirmed that her panic attacks and fears of loss of control were triggered when she felt she had to yield to others and was angry about this submission. Although Ms. DDD remained off antidepressant medication, her intense reaction and its transference manifestations provided valuable information in understanding her panic symptoms. Her symptoms responded to psychotherapy and a minimal dose of as-needed benzodiazepines.

The Transitional Object Function of Medication in Anxious Patients

Medication functioning as a transitional object was discussed in some detail in chapter 4. In this view (Hausner, 1985), the medication can take on the meaning of a safety object, symbolically averting a separation. Fearful dependency and associated separation fears are common in panic and other anxiety patients, who are particularly susceptible to experiencing the medication in this way. This can be an aspect of the placebo function in medication, perhaps contributing to the high rate of placebo response found for panic patients. Panic patients will often carry medication with them "just in case," thus providing a feeling of safety beyond that from taking the medication. This safety aspect can disrupt patients' ability to taper off medication even when appropriate. In chapter 4, the case of Ms. T described how medication, like other objects of the patient's parents and therapist, provided protection from separation fears. Ultimately, exploration of these objects is important because attachment to them can be a means of avoiding addressing intrapsychic threats.

For example, Ms. EEE, a 35-year-old woman who suffered from panic disorder and occasional depressive symptoms, expressed unwillingness to attempt to taper her 2-mg daily dose of lorazepam, despite a good response to venlafaxine. Ms. EEE described a series of traumatic disruptions early in life when her wealthy parents would leave for extended periods on vacation. In addition, when her parents were at home, she felt that they were not responsive when she needed help. For instance, she described a sleepover in which she was injured, ultimately requiring stitches, but her parents left it to the other family to manage the situation, despite the patient's pleas. Anger at her parents intermixed in this patient with fearful dependency in the cycle described earlier. In exploration of the attachment to her medication other transitional objects emerged.

Ms. EEE: It's not just medication I'm attached to. I have two teddy bears in my bed I've had since childhood. I take them everywhere I go. In fact, my last boyfriend was very upset by them. I don't like to think about being without them.

Therapist: What happens when you do?

Ms. EEE: I feel terrified. Even talking about it now feels very scary. They've always been important to me.

Therapist: I wonder if they were important in protecting you from separation fears when your parents were away.

Ms. EEE: And even when they were there. Because even then I felt like they sometimes weren't emotionally present.

Therapist: Well, I think we should explore these fears further.

Ms. EEE: As long as I don't have to give them up.

The degree of anxiety Ms. EEE experienced in discussing this topic was striking. Exploring associated fears of loss and emptiness, as well as her frightening anger at her parents, helped to better approach the patient's attachment to medication.

Anxiety Disorders and Pregnancy

As noted earlier, pregnancy involves multiple issues for patients with anxiety disorders. Pregnancy can trigger fears of loss of control, damage to the body, aggression toward the child, and loss of the child role. Psychopharmacological treatment during pregnancy is a complex issue, with recommendations against the use of benzodiazepines, particularly in the first trimester, and guarded use of certain antidepressants. Due to underlying fantasies, patients with anxiety may be particularly frightened of potential harm to the fetus from medication.

Ms. FFF was a 30-year-old woman who presented with severe panic symptoms and generalized anxiety disorder, with particular worries about her health. Despite being married and planning to have a child, she was in close contact with her parents regarding her health concerns. She would regularly inform them about her symptoms, review the comments of her doctors, and discuss how to proceed with her care. This advice seeking was part of a more general tendency to get help from her parents about many matters in her life, including clothing, decorating tips, and relationship conflicts.

This relationship appeared to have a long history, with her mother focused on her doing things "the right way" socially from early in her life, although she felt her mother was unable to help her with bullying in her seventh grade class. Health concerns were exacerbated in eighth grade, when her mother developed colon cancer requiring surgery and chemotherapy. Ms. FFF and her parents were also traumatized by a near fatal bout of appendicitis when she went to college. Currently, Ms. FFF felt pressured to submit to her mother's views and to bring her worries to her and greatly feared the loss of this caretaking relationship.

In the setting of plans for having her first child, Ms. FFF developed an exacerbation of her severe panic and comorbid depression. She was started on sertraline with resolution of symptoms, but subsequently was frightened by the idea of getting pregnant on the medication. Exploration revealed a series of concerns about having a baby. Ms. FFF feared losing her dependency on her parents and was frightened about being the mother rather than the child. In addition, it emerged that behind her submission to her parents was an intense anger at her mother's intrusiveness that she found threatening, and she feared this anger would also develop toward her child.

Ms. FFF's conflict became focused on the medication. In accord with a view of the medication as an object (discussed in chapter 4), the medication became the maternal object, which she needed and feared giving up and yet resented because of her feelings of dependency and experience of intrusion. In addition, she feared feeling guilty should anything happen to her child from medication, which was linked to her anger at her future child for forcing her to give up her own childlike position.

Ms. FFF's pregnancy efforts were delayed several months as she struggled with her fantasies about the medication and pregnancy and after a failed effort to discontinue the medication. Ultimately, as these various fears were explored, Ms. FFF understood that her conflicts about pregnancy were being displaced onto the medication. She recognized the exaggerated and conflicted fear she felt about "losing" her parents, as well as the threat of her anger at parent and future child alike. These realizations helped her to understand her anxiety and also to make a decision to proceed with the pregnancy on medication. No problems were evident at the birth of her child.

Combined Treatment of Obsessive–Compulsive Disorder

Obsessive–compulsive disorder (OCD) was an important area of clinical observation and theorizing for early psychoanalysts. In a psychodynamic formulation of OCD, patients are viewed as struggling with aggressive or sexual fantasies and feelings that are considered unacceptable to a severe superego, and they fear loss of control of these feelings. The danger the patient feels is intensified by a regression or persistence of an early stage of ego development, in which thoughts were felt to be equivalent to an action. Defenses are triggered in an attempt to cope with these wishes, such as undoing via compulsive behaviors designed to make restitution for the aggressive and sexual wishes, and intellectualization to minimize frightening feelings.

OCD symptoms can be understood as a compromise formation between aggressive and sexual wishes and the attempt to undo them with penitential acts to ward off guilt and anxiety. Freud (1909b), for example, described the case of a patient who developed a compulsive symptom of moving a stone back and forth into the road to cope with aggressive wishes and ambivalence toward a woman (thinking her carriage would hit the stone) and the need to undo the fantasy of damage. More recent psychoanalytic thinkers view the aggression and guilt as resulting from the experience of critical or neglectful parents (Brandchaft, 2001; Meares, 2001). In this formulation, obsessional symptoms represent efforts to control the threat of disrupted attachments to significant others.

Psychoanalysts have been less focused on OCD in recent years, in part due to the demonstrated efficacy of other approaches (cognitive behavioral therapy and some antidepressants) in treating OCD and evidence of a biological origin in many cases (Esman, 1989, 2001). A combined treatment of OCD is common, and psychodynamic approaches, though not systematically studied, can aid patients through a focus on the meaning of symptoms (Gabbard, 2000, 2001). Fears of loss of control and feelings of shame can arise in the context of exploring symptoms and prescribing medication. The psychoanalytic therapist's nonjudgmental stance can help patients to feel safer about revealing obsessions and compulsions and taking medication. Transference and countertransference fantasies can be identified to aid patients with problems in interpersonal relationships secondary to OCD.

Leahy, McGinn, Busch, and Milrod (2005) describe the case of a patient, Linda, a 40-year-old single woman whose long-standing rituals of checking the locks and gas and repeated hand-washing had increasingly interfered with her life in recent months. She would also read her horoscope repeatedly, looking for clues about future dangers. These symptoms had worsened in the context of deepening intimacy with her boyfriend, with whom she was considering marriage. Alongside her rituals, she developed obsessional preoccupations that her boyfriend was interested in another woman, with whom he would become involved and then leave her.

Efforts to explore the functions of her symptoms were initially stymied by the degree of her anxious preoccupation. She expressed fear about taking medication, with a worry that others would see her as "crazy," but exploration of feelings of shame relieved her concern. A trial of sertraline significantly reduced her symptoms, allowing further psychodynamic exploration.

Linda described problems growing up with a father who demanded a high level of academic and professional achievement, although she felt ultimately unable to gain his love. Her father was often distant, and there were suggestions that he was involved in affairs with other women. She saw her mother, an anxious and intrusive woman, as incompetent, and she viewed herself as her mother's caretaker. Many of her rituals and obsessions were understood to be efforts to control her fears of rejection, intrusiveness, and anger in the context of her increasing involvement with her boyfriend. Study of her horoscope focused on fantasies that she would be able to determine whether he would reject her. The identification of the meaning of her symptoms combined with medication to further diminish her obsessions and compulsions.

Countertransference Issues With Anxious Patients

Patients with anxiety disorders can induce several countertransference reactions that may affect the use of medication by psychiatrists. Anxious patients can create anxious feelings in the therapist, which could lead to overuse of medication. In these instances, the therapist may be inadvertently, perhaps unconsciously, blocking the emergence of feelings and fantasies that the patient (and perhaps the therapist) find to be frightening. In addition to reacting to the anxiety, therapists should be alert to frustration with patients stemming from their dependency and difficulty taking autonomous steps. Therapists may respond to this frustration by overmedicating in an attempt to eliminate these conflicts or undermedicating as an unconscious expression of their irritation. Subtle or direct criticism or angry expressions will confirm patients' expectations of attack and disrupt the therapeutic alliance.

When prescribing medication, therapists can become frustrated by patients' anxious preoccupations about medications, which sometimes require very slow increases in dosage to aid patients in tolerance. Patients may see medication as representing the damaging hurtful other that needs to be warded off; therapists will sometimes become frustrated with patients' views of the medication, and thereby the therapist, as hurtful or damaging. Therapists should be alert to these reactions because they can provide clues to communicate to patients in a helpful way about factors that lead them to fear or struggle with the prescription of medication.

In the case of Ms. FFF, the patient appeared to be ready to proceed with her pregnancy efforts after addressing a series of fears about continuing the medication. However, Ms. FFF stated that her mother had raised new objections, after speaking with a doctor friend of hers who viewed the medication as unsafe. Ms. FFF felt more time would be needed to get a handle on this doctor's concerns, and her mother felt it was important for the therapist to respond to these issues.

At this point, the therapist became aware of frustration at the patient for this new anxiety about medication and pregnancy. On looking at this reaction, he noted that one component was the narcissistic injury of feeling that his view was not good enough and that another doctor's opinion would trump his. More strongly, however, he felt the urge to tell Ms. FFF, "Look. Just get on with it. That's enough objections already."

This thought helped the therapist to understand more about how the patient induced controlling behavior from others. Her anxious preoccupations and indecisiveness led her mother to intervene more authoritatively with her. This helped to maintain the dependent relationship: Despite Ms. FFF's frustration with her mother's intervention, she often provoked it by presenting herself as incompetent. Communicating this concept to her not only helped her to proceed with pregnancy, but also aided her in examining the ways her behavior exacerbated problems with her mother.

9

Complex Cases

In this chapter, we turn to complex cases. We will discuss a number of common clinical scenarios that are particularly challenging when engaged in combined treatment. These include managing suicidal patients, repeated symptom recurrence, treatment-resistant cases, chronically noncompliant patients, and substance abuse. Rather than focusing on technical aspects of pharmacological treatment of these cases, the chapter will describe how a combined approach provides additional tools for helping such patients. We will also discuss the question of whether medication can interfere with integration (Swoiskin, 2001) through a contemporary lens.

THE SUICIDAL PATIENT

No event is more traumatic for the clinician than the suicide of one of his or her patients (Tillman, 2006). While suicide is a rare event—in the United States the annual incidence of suicide is estimated at 10.7 for every 100,000 persons—suicide attempts and suicidal ideation are relatively common and estimated at approximately 0.7 and 5.6% of the general U.S. population per year, respectively (American Psychiatric Association, 2000). Suicide assessment scales have been developed for research purposes but do not have predictive validity for routine clinical use. The identification of known risk factors (for example, major depression, substance use, psychotic disorder, hopelessness) can alert the clinician to relative risk, but the rarity of suicide makes it impossible to predict who will die by suicide. A further complication is that some patients chronically engage in self-injurious behavior or harbor wishes to be dead. The confluence of these factors can contribute to therapeutic nihilism or complacency with this population. Countertransference factors, including hateful feelings toward the suicidal patient (Maltsberger & Buie, 1974), can further complicate treatment.

Nondynamic psychotherapies (interpersonal therapy and cognitive behavior therapy) have proven efficacy in the treatment of specific disorders (major depression, for example) associated with suicide, and modest evidence exists for the role of psychodynamic treatment in borderline personality disorder in diminishing self-injurious behavior (American Psychiatric Association, 2000). However, Hendin et al. (2006) observe that most clinicians treat suicidal patients in an open-ended eclectic psychotherapy (i.e., one that incorporates cognitive behavior and interpersonal techniques along with a reliance on psychodynamic principles). The more seriously disturbed suicidal patient tends to receive medication in combination with this open-ended psychotherapeutic approach. Their research project endeavored to identify patterns of problems in working with suicidal patients in an open-ended therapy. Data were collected from therapists of 36 patients who had died by suicide. While limited by the retrospective nature of the study, many of their observations have direct relevance to the issue of combined treatment in this population.

One critical finding was the lack of communication between therapists when treatment was split between a social worker or psychologist and a psychiatrist. Hendin et al. (2006) described one case as illustrative: A man with recurrent depression and suicidal ideation of many years' duration was urged by his social worker therapist to discuss his medication noncompliance with his psychiatrist, but the therapist did not contact the psychiatrist. The patient often expressed suicidal thoughts (to both therapist and psychiatrist) with an explicit plan, but asserted he would not harm himself while his parents were alive.

Nine days prior to the patient's suicide and coincident with his mother becoming increasingly impaired due to bipolar illness, the patient told the psychiatrist that he had looked at a gun in a store and thought of putting it in his mouth. The psychiatrist sent him home reassured by his promise that he would not harm himself. One day prior to his death, the man met with his therapist and again voiced active suicidal ideation. The therapist offered him more frequent visits and phone support. He killed himself the next day. The authors raise the possibility that a more proactive intervention might have taken place had the therapist and psychiatrist had direct communication. This could have facilitated a heightened awareness of the role of medication noncompliance increasing the patient's suicidal risk.

While split treatment created potential problems in communication with the treatment team, 80% of cases involved a single practitioner, suggesting the importance of other considerations. In almost half the cases, therapists permitted patients or their relatives to control the treatment. Frequently, the therapist feared upsetting an already fragile patient. Of particular relevance was the finding that in 25% of the cases, the patients' wish for control led them to decide their own medication regimen. In each case, psychotherapy was compromised due to mood-related impairment in ego functioning, but therapists felt helpless and went along even in cases where patients stopped taking their medication completely.

This problem was closely related to another: In almost half the patients, symptoms were either untreated or undertreated. This included a number of patients suffering from anxiety prior to their suicide and a small number who had psychotic symptoms that were undiagnosed. Untreated substance abuse was a major problem in about one-third of the population.

A last critical problem area was that therapists did not recognize the meanings of patients' communications. While this did not exclusively pertain to the meaning of medication, in one example, a bipolar patient with a history of suicidal behavior called his therapist asking for reassurance that his ingestion of double the dose of his medicine was not really a suicide attempt but accidental. The therapist reassured him. He killed himself the following week.

These findings suggest that, while a single practitioner eliminates one critical problem—that of inadequate communication between therapists, the prescribing therapist may be particularly vulnerable to not adequately addressing patients' acting out around medication. This is sobering in that over 80% of these patients were being seen at least weekly and over 30% were being seen three times per week. Among the authors' conclusions is the following:

> Patients' control over medication presents a particularly difficult dilemma in treating suicidal patients. Although confronting patients about control over or discontinuation of medication carries the risk that they will terminate treatment, therapists' passive permissiveness in regard to patients' (or their relatives') attempts to control the treatment commonly engenders anxiety, anger, and disconnection in suicidal patients. Explicitly exploring the patient's feelings about medication noncompliance is essential. (p. 71)

The depressed suicidal patient who is incapable of taking potentially lifesaving medication as prescribed likely suffers from severe state-related impairments in ego functioning. If the patient is unable to use the therapist as an auxiliary ego, more drastic steps, including hospitalization, need to be considered. Even when medication compliance is not a major issue, treating this patient population can be challenging, as evidenced by the case of Ms. GGG.

Ms. GGG, a 50-year-old married woman, was referred for psychopharmacological consultation by her analyst for assessment of depressive symptoms, triggered by news that her mother's cancer had spread and was untreatable. The consultant noted the presence of symptoms consistent with major depression along with significant anxiety, though no overt panic. She had no suicidal ideation on presentation. She said she had one or two glasses of wine per night. She complained of a long-standing terror of being alone, feelings of emptiness, and emotional instability consistent with the referring analyst's impression of borderline pathology.

The patient also described a tumultuous relationship with a narcissistic mother (an actress) who often failed in her ability to empathize with the patient's inner state. For example, when the patient told the mother that she herself had been diagnosed with cancer, the mother asked if she planned to get a wig to deal with the effects of chemotherapy. Her parents divorced when she was 4 years old, at which time she moved far away from her father.

Ms. GGG was started on citalopram and began to notice an improvement in mood and anxiety symptoms by the second month. However, her mother's death from cancer during the third month of medication (and seventh month of analysis) triggered a significant deterioration in mood. She felt guilty about having revealed her mother's cruelty (experiencing this as a betrayal) and anticipating a large inheritance that she did not feel she deserved. She experienced further guilt in having withheld from her therapists that she had been abusing oxycodone intermittently for years and her use had escalated significantly in recent months.

Ms. GGG developed suicidal ideation, without any conscious intent, that included thoughts about not getting out of the way of an oncoming bus and wondering about "going over" her terrace. A further important trigger to her drop in mood was her growing attachment to her analyst, who represented a good mother but who would soon be leaving the patient for her summer vacation. The analyst contacted the pharmacotherapist to inform him of Ms. GGG's deteriorating condition.

Analyst: I'm worried about Ms. GGG. Her guilt has a delusional quality with her expectation that her mother will punish her. Anticipating the inheritance, she's become convinced her mother will never forgive her for being a bad daughter.

Pharmacotherapist: How concerned are you about her safety?

Analyst: She has active suicidal ideation but denies any intent to harm herself. But last week she ingested cough medicine with codeine and hit her head on the table, requiring stitches. She expressed more indifference about hurting herself rather than a wish to be dead.

Pharmacotherapist: Clearly this is an unstable situation. I'd like to evaluate her on an urgent basis and figure out whether she can safely be treated on an ambulatory basis or not. She may need ECT. I'll also ask her to have her husband come along so that I can have additional input from him and have him as an ally.

Analyst: Ms. GGG doesn't want to go to the hospital. She's terrified of hospitals, given her own and her mother's experiences with cancer. It's come up in our sessions this week.

Pharmacotherapist: I assume that the fact it's come up in your work is an indication of how out of control she feels.

Analyst: I agree.

Two days later, the patient met with the pharmacotherapist, at which time Ms. GGG was ruminating about an upcoming date for her mother's ashes to be spread—an experience she felt she could not tolerate and one she believed her mother would never forgive her for missing. She expressed the delusional belief that her mother was angry with her, as evidenced by the fact that she had had only one dream in which her mother figured since her death. The patient, while guilt ridden, did not feel she deserved death, nor did she have a reunion fantasy with the mother whose wrath she feared. Careful exploration of her suicidal thoughts revealed occasional thoughts of a "dramatic" nature to jump out a window while she asserted, "I wouldn't take it into my own hands to make it happen."

Given the mother's histrionic tendencies, both therapists construed the dramatic nature of her fantasy as a worrisome and potentially deadly identification with her mother. Her husband felt that Ms. GGG was "not herself." After explaining to the patient and her husband his reasons for concern, the pharmacotherapist recommended hospitalization to manage a psychotic depression complicated by substance abuse. Both patient and husband were adamantly opposed to hospitalization and, without the husband's support and without the patient being actively suicidal, he moved to "Plan B."

Pharmacotherapist: We will need to see in the days and weeks ahead if ongoing treatment outside the hospital will work for you. I am going to make a change in your medication that I'll discuss shortly, but first we need to discuss your safety.

Ms. GGG: I don't think I would do anything to hurt myself.

Pharmacotherapist: Yet you're having thoughts about jumping out a window or off a balcony.

Ms. GGG: I would never do that. It would hurt my husband.

Pharmacotherapist: How will you manage if your feelings change? What can you do?

Ms. GGG: I would call you or my analyst. But I think I'll be OK.

Pharmacotherapist: Let's move to Plan B: That will include our having a lot more contact over the next few days and weeks.

The pharmacotherapist instituted a change in medication (from citalopram to venlafaxine and risperidone) and spoke with Ms. GGG's analyst about the treatment plan and his concerns for her safety. He failed to follow up on Ms. GGG's opiate abuse—an oversight on his part. However, the following week, she guiltily confessed to her analyst that she had withheld an alcohol problem that included hard liquor and wine over many years. While this no doubt was another worrisome part of the clinical picture, her capacity to engage her analyst honestly helped to mobilize the treatment team to introduce Alcoholics Anonymous as an additional part of her treatment.

Over the next several weeks, her depressive symptoms slowly remitted. She struggled with her addictive behavior but moved toward abstinence, and her suicidal ideation markedly shifted from thoughts about being dead to wanting to be out of emotional pain. Even passive suicidal thoughts were attenuated: from wanting to sleep forever to wanting to sleep to escape her pain. The control of her severe depressive symptoms with pharmacotherapy created an optimal foundation for subsequent intensive psychotherapy that spanned 6 years with no recurrence of suicidal ideation. This case illustrates the importance of a collaborative approach by the treating therapists, the need for aggressive pharmacologic management of depressive symptoms, and the value of ongoing vigilance about substance abuse.

TREATMENT-RESISTANT CASES: MOOD DISORDERS AND PERSONALITY

Resistance within a psychoanalytic frame of reference refers to a dynamic state within the patient who fends off the therapist's efforts through various defensive means. An extreme version of this is the stalemated clinical situation, the term itself implying a dynamic, albeit stalled, state of affairs between patient and therapist. Within the psychiatric literature, resistant or refractory illness is not consistently defined (Fava & Davidson, 1996; Guscott & Grof, 1991; Sackheim, 2001). However, it typically refers to an illness that is nonresponsive or incompletely responsive to one or more standard treatments. A dynamic meaning does not apply. Clinicians are cautioned to look for coexisting disorders that can interfere with adequate treatment and alert to the possibility of "pseudoresistance" due to undertreatment with medication (Sackheim, 2001).

The psychodynamic clinician will attempt to assess both dynamic and nondynamic aspects of treatment resistance as well as the possible relationship between the two. As discussed in chapter 2, teasing these factors apart can be difficult. At times, it may be useful to consider resistance along a medical model; for example, pneumonias can be antibiotic resistant and depressions can be drug resistant. At other times, the resistance may be more usefully conceptualized along psychodynamic lines; for example, a guilt-ridden patient repeatedly undermines the treatment as an expression of a negative therapeutic reaction. The clinician will attempt to evaluate the plausibility of the different causes of resistance.

Wylie and Wylie (1995), employing an interactional model, observe that dynamic and nondynamic aspects are frequently interwoven. The fact that the boundaries between the two can be difficult to delineate adds further to the clinical challenge. Paradigmatic of this challenge is working with depressed patients who also have personality disorders. Howland and Thase (2005) observe that a large number of individuals with chronic and refractory depression suffer with personality disorders.

The clinician's approach will depend upon his theoretical perspective about the relationship between the conditions he is treating. For example, Akiskal and colleagues (Akiskal, Hirshfeld, & Yerevanian, 1983; Akiskal et al., 1985) are major proponents of the view that personality characteristics can represent mild (subclinical) or alternate (spectrum) manifestations of an underlying biologically determined mood disorder. They cite research that supports a neurobiological continuity between many personality disorders and depression (abnormal sleep architecture with shortened REM latency).

Some antidepressant drug studies show a reversal or alleviation of characterologic problems (Akiskal, 2005). Neurobiological and genetic studies also suggest interesting continuities between depression and personality. Howland and Thase (2005) summarize the influence of polymorphisms of the serotonin transporter gene on depression and its treatment. Presence of the short allele influences symptom presentation (more depressive symptoms and suicidality in relation to stressful life events) and is associated with the personality traits of neuroticism and negative emotionality. The long allele predicts a better response to SSRIs. Howland and Thase speculate that stress responsiveness may be genetically determined in some people and reflects a common vulnerability for depression and personality disorders. Some patients may be susceptible to getting more depressed with a given stress but also predisposed to enter stressful life circumstances, setting up a vicious cycle (Thase & Howland, 1994).

In addition to neurobiological and genetic continuities between mood disorders and personality, the psychodynamic clinician will also consider the psychological links between the two (Blatt, 2004). The fact that such continuities exist, while not surprising, reveals how complicated the effort to distinguish the neurobiological "obstruction" from the dynamic "resistance" can be (Wylie & Wylie, 1995). Writing as psychiatrist and psychoanalyst, Friedman (1991) illustrates the challenge and utility of such an effort. He made a series of observations confined to a difficult-to-treat group of patients who had severe mood disorders in addition to masochistic character pathology.

While the masochistic character has been abandoned as a diagnostic category in the DSM-IV (American Psychiatric Association, 1994), it continues to be a useful conceptualization for many clinicians—a fact supported by its inclusion in the recently published *Psychodynamic Diagnostic Manual* (PDM Task Force, 2006). Friedman's primary thesis is that a large number of chronically depressed patients have comorbid masochistic pathology. This subgroup is characterized by a suboptimal response to treatment of the depressive illness with pharmacotherapy. He argues that these patients require the thoughtful integration of both pharmacologic and psychotherapeutic approaches in order to achieve a good outcome.

Friedman (1991) urges caution in making a diagnosis of masochism when a patient is in a clinical depression. While analysts emphasize the importance of the underlying character structure, Friedman observes that, in a depressed state, a patient who presents appearing blatantly masochistic can have substantial relief of these symptoms with adequate treatment of the depressive illness. Without longitudinal data and possibly corroborative data from a relative, the clinician must use caution concluding that significant masochistic pathology exists in the midst of a depressive illness. The patient must be observed through treatment of the mood disorder to see how his character is modified.

For example, Friedman presents a case of a woman who in a helpless and self-denigrating manner lamented her incapacity to manage relationships. The initial impression of a masochistic character shifted, upon more careful questioning, to the diagnosis of major depression characterized by suicidal thoughts, sleep disturbance, pessimism, loss of sexual desire, and weight gain. Treatment of the mood symptoms resulted in the "entire panoply of apparently severe character symptoms melting away" (1991, p. 18). Depression can be overlooked when a patient presents dramatically with self-defeating traits. In these situations, a sadomasochistic transference can evolve, with the undiagnosed depressive condition left untreated.

The clinician must also be careful not to miss the diagnosis of masochism. Friedman (1991) gives an example of a man with a long-standing history of depression who repeatedly accepted treatment for depression, only to become noncompliant after responding to medication. He would typically blame the clinician for his relapse, feeling like a victim. It was only after the therapist noted the patient's repeated self-defeating behavior in relation to treatment as well as in major areas of his personal life that he was able to address this problem as distinct from his depressive illness. This approach succeeded in helping the patient stay on maintenance medication after a suicide attempt and to engage in an insight-oriented psychotherapy to address a self-destructive pattern that permeated his life.

Friedman (1991) observes the essential continuities between depression and masochism from a psychodynamic perspective. In particular, self-directed aggression figures prominently in both clinical states. For Friedman, masochistic patients are a subgroup of chronic depressives characterized by hostility and helplessness. The core masochistic fantasy is a way to cope with and control painful feelings, especially depression. Friedman also provides a clinical pearl: For the masochist, the persistent experience of pain is a key feature deemed essential for psychological equilibrium. Whereas the clinician will have as a goal the remission of symptoms of major depression, the patient unconsciously motivated to be in a state of controlled misery will often not be able to tolerate getting better. As indicated in the preceding vignette, such patients will often stop their medication prematurely or end their therapy. Anticipation of these risks can equip the therapist to better meet these challenges.

How do Akiskal and Friedman compare in their theoretical approach and clinical formulation? Both caution the clinician not to make a diagnosis of character disorder in the setting of a significant mood disorder so as not to undertreat the latter condition and possibly misdiagnose significant character pathology during a state of illness. However, Akiskal (2005) sees the characterologic symptoms as derivative of the mood disorder. Hence, he emphasizes the role of medication as primary and psychosocial interventions as secondary. Akiskal (2005) states, "True, affectively ill patients often harbor self-defeating thoughts, but in practice these are best regarded as an integral part of the illness" (p. xiv). He is particularly critical of the notion of patients resisting. In this way he parts ways with Friedman and other psychodynamic clinicians who assert the ongoing value and necessity of a psychodynamic perspective as a way of understanding and helping this patient population. Masochistic pathology overlaps depressive illness but is also distinct from it, though the lines of demarcation are often unclear.

Ms. W, previously discussed in chapter 4, was referred for outpatient treatment, having been hospitalized after ingesting 12 mg of lorazepam in a suicide attempt. She had received 12 ECTs for a psychotic depression characterized by profound guilt that she linked to encouraging her sister to smoke (and hence putting her at risk for cancer and death) and feeling attracted to girls. During an extended consultation, the therapist found the patient withdrawn and guarded, though she reassured him she would not harm herself again. However, she believed she deserved to die for her "crimes" and saw this criminal activity as the basis for intense self-hatred. She felt she had a "duty" to hurt herself for her crimes. The therapist contacted the hospital psychiatrist and expressed the concern that the patient continued to be severely depressed, even though neurovegetative symptoms were no longer present. She received six more ECTs and was then discharged on maintenance medication (sertraline and fluphenazine).

At the beginning of her psychotherapy following discharge, she said very little about her childhood experience, other than having been "well-raised" by her parents and being burdened by guilt in relation to her sister, who was 4 years younger. As the treatment got under way, a clearer picture emerged of a woman with long-standing masochistic traits embedded in a borderline personality. Her sense of "badness" was not confined to the state of depression; it was a core part of her identity. Early on she said, "I am either an empty shell or I am evil. There is nothing else." Slowly a picture of a devastating childhood emerged, characterized by severe physical abuse by her mother and a fear of disintegrating when looking into her mother's eyes, either due to her mother's rage or as a reflection of her own. She had marked difficulty tolerating the kindness and support of her therapist because she felt unworthy of love.

Over the course of a 12-year treatment, the therapist repeatedly struggled with her entrenched suffering and need to suffer—at times considering the picture one of residual depression warranting more aggressive medication management. Sometimes, the therapist viewed it through a psychodynamic lens and at other times considered the interaction between the two. Multiple medication trials in conjunction with a twice weekly psychotherapy permitted Ms. W to work full time and stabilize her marriage. The shift to a complex medication regimen (lamotrigine, olanzapine, escitalopram) took place after an intensification of symptoms of depression that appeared triggered by a deepening of the psychotherapy. The patient felt herself sinking into "quicksand" and "the abyss" as she made contact with her murderous rage toward her mother.

Ms. W: I feel like killing her … and myself. I don't want to be buried near her! How can I say that to a priest?

Therapist: It's very painful for you to get in touch with your murderous feelings toward your mother. I think you must have been terrified as a child—of your mother's rage and the rage you felt toward her.

Ms. W: I was mortified. Her eyes were terrifying. I thought I would die … at times I felt I would be better off being dead. (Becomes sad.) I'm afraid of my anger—I fear I'll disintegrate if I get in touch with it. I have no sense of self.

Therapist: I think you fear disintegrating in part because you turn the anger you feel onto yourself. You didn't experience your mother's cruelty as abuse. In your effort to extract love, you told yourself that her verbal attacks and beatings were acts of love that you deserved for being a bad girl. Self-flagellation has been a way to stay attached to your mother.

Ms. W: If I think about my mother's badness instead of my own I fear disintegrating. I know now from our work together that she was very ill and maltreated me. But, at the same time, it's very hard for me to keep that in mind without becoming terrified I'll be destroyed.

Therapist: I think the medication will help to reduce your depression. I also think that the strong emotions that are being stirred up, while you fear being destroyed by them, will ultimately help you to feel more alive. I think you have enormous sadness—grief—inside of you about the horrific childhood you had, not just emptiness or rage.

Ms. W: I have never been able to feel sad for myself.

After years of work with Ms. W with multiple medication adjustments and psychotherapy, the therapist suggested a trial of intensifying the psychotherapy from two times a week to three times per week. The initial resistance was that she was unworthy of the therapist's care and she already felt like a burden. Examining the developmental underpinnings of this view led her to intensify the treatment and begin a process of mourning that at times felt overwhelming to her, but was distinctly different from being depressed. Guilt, which had been a tenacious symptom in her state of depression and characterologically, gave way to a greater acceptance of herself as having goodness inside her and hence being able to receive goodness from others, including the therapist. She gradually became more comfortable with her own aggression and began to feel, as she was approaching her sixth decade of life, that she existed for the first time in her life.

In this case, there was a significant overlap between Ms. W's masochistic symptomatology and her depressive illness. When neurovegetative symptoms emerged or her sense of badness seemed intractable, the therapist considered more aggressive pharmacotherapy. By working to stabilize her mood pharmacologically, the therapist was able to help the patient tolerate the painful psychotherapeutic work of mourning.

Complex cases involving mood and personality are not confined to depressive illness. There has been significant interest and controversy in the literature about the relationship between bipolar illness and borderline personality. There are varying degrees of comorbidity between these conditions depending on how broadly bipolar illness is defined (Bieling & MacQueen, 2005). Drug studies support the utility of mood stabilizers for borderline patients with and without bipolar illness (Noblett & Cocarro, 2005; Preston et al., 2004). However, in a large longitudinal study, Gunderson et al. (2006) found only a modest association exists between these two conditions and concluded that a "strong spectrum relationship with bipolar disorder is extremely unlikely" (p. 1177). Their findings do not support the hypothesis, championed by Akiskal and colleagues (1983), that borderline personality is a variant of bipolar disorder. Furthermore,

> Despite the fact that these disorders only co-occur in 10–25% of patients with either disorder, it has become unusual for patients with borderline personality disorder not to have been diagnosed with bipolar disorder, usually bipolar II disorder. The absence of a strong association between borderline personality disorder and bipolar disorder indicates that clinicians should attend to the differences. ... omitting the borderline personality diagnosis diverts therapeutic efforts away from psychosocial interventions that can often make a remarkable difference. (p. 1177)

According to Gunderson et al. (2006), affective instability of borderline personality should not be conceptualized as a bipolar type instability for most patients. Clinicians should not lose sight of what is distinctive about borderline patients. However, when the conditions do co-occur, treatment can be very challenging.

Told she had the "evil eye" by a psychotic mother, Ms. HHH suffered with a severe, rapidly cycling bipolar illness and borderline personality that would emerge more clearly when her bipolar disorder was under control (characterized by emptiness and identity diffusion). When depressed, she would become psychotic and suicidal, convinced that she looked and smelled like her father, whom she despised. Her manic states were often characterized by irritability, paranoia, and increased energy. She would impulsively spend money during these periods, purchasing things that she neither enjoyed nor wanted. When the high periods remitted, she would find herself left with "crap" along with a substantial debt. The "crap" would include clothes she disliked (even when making the purchases) and various cleaning supplies for her home.

Over years of treatment, Ms. HHH and the therapist came to understand her increased spending as a clear expression of mania, while the purchases themselves had profound symbolic significance. Having been told she was evil and ugly from a young age, Ms. HHH chronically felt unworthy of love and unloving. Her manic purchases expressed core conflicts around her identity: "I am an ugly person so I should buy clothes I find ugly." "I am evil inside and dirty. I should try to be clean."

The striking absence of heightened self-esteem during these periods, along with the masochistic quality of the pleasure she had, helped Ms. HHH and her therapist understand how her bipolar illness and personality difficulties were simultaneously expressed in her increased spending. Aggressive pharmacotherapy to stabilize her mood and an extended period of intensive psychotherapy helped Ms. HHH to own her murderous rage toward her parents, mourn her childhood, and develop an enduring capacity for self-love. This would not have been possible without attending to the bipolar illness and her borderline personality, as well as the intersection of the two.

CHRONIC NONCOMPLIANCE WITH MEDICATION

Chronic noncompliance with medication creates a vicious cycle that, left uninterrupted, can result in treatment failure or chronic sadomasochistic transferences. Mintz (2002) encourages a systematic focus on the meaning of medication as a way of managing the resistance to optimizing care. It is also helpful to consider what the patient is trying to create within the transference–countertransference through noncompliance.

While we speak of "compliance," we eschew the therapist assuming an authoritarian attitude. As discussed in chapter 3, the patient should be as involved as possible in the decision-making process about medication, taking into account ego deficits that may be state related (mood, anxiety, or psychotic symptoms) and personality issues. Some patients will struggle with their need for medication when in an acute state of illness and, when improved, will again struggle with issues that may or may not be related to their initial reluctance to take medication. By avoiding the pejorative connotation of "noncompliance," the therapist is more likely to maintain an open curiosity as to the transference issues about taking the medicine. As was discussed with the suicidal patient, therapists can inadvertently fail to confront patients who are acting in a self-injurious way by not taking medication. While state-related anxieties (i.e., related to the acute illness being medicated) will sometimes cause noncompliance, underlying personality issues, which can evoke strong countertransference reactions, are likely to be factors in chronic disorders.

Mr. III, a 40-year-old married teacher of learning-disabled children, came for consultation in a markedly agitated, "paranoid" state, saying, "Medication is requisite." Pressured in his speech and irritable, he spoke of a chronically stressful life and an escalating feeling of rage that "the world is against me," while at other moments reflecting "my reactions occur in the absence of stimuli." He was mildly thought-disordered with an overly intellectualized manner of speech, reflecting his use of obsessional defenses to bind his anxiety. While acknowledging racing thoughts, poor sleep, and irritability, he simultaneously experienced intense low moods, low energy, and poor concentration. The initial impression was of a mixed bipolar state.

Mr. III reported long-standing difficulties due to an arrogant attitude and controlling behavior that were deemed disrespectful, condescending, and insubordinate. He compulsively tried to help those in need—an endeavor that often sounded grandiose. He grew up poor in a strict household and recalled his father often yelling at his mother, a behavior he now saw replayed in his own marriage in ways that threatened it. As a young child, he was frequently teased, bullied, and beat up because of his short stature. The therapist entertained the possibility of narcissistic and paranoid personality traits, though it was also possible that he was chronically unstable due to an untreated bipolar illness.

During an 18-month period, successive medication trials were attempted. These included mood stabilizers (valproic acid, lithium carbonate, and lamotrigine) and atypical antipsychotics (quetiapine and risperidone). Mr. III was most comfortable with risperidone, a drug that he felt reduced his paranoia. However, efforts to optimize his treatment repeatedly failed because he expressed dissatisfaction due to side effects or persistent symptoms. He would often act as his own doctor, stopping medication on his own.

Finally, the therapist decided to move to a trial of escitalopram with risperidone to manage worsening depression 4 months after Mr. III's father's sudden death. The patient "in error" took double the dose of escitalopram and became markedly agitated to the point that he felt he was going to hurt himself. Even with low doses, he had restlessness like he was "jumping out of [his] skin." He rejected escitalopram after that. Lorazepam was added on an urgent basis, and he was encouraged to take it regularly, while monitoring for sedation. Within a day or so, he felt much calmer, though "drugged," at which point the therapist encouraged him to reduce the dose a small amount. Although at first he thought of the lorazepam as a lifesaver, he quickly shifted his focus to problems he felt it created.

Mr. III: (angrily) I am deeply depressed and I think it's because of the lorazepam. I know it can cause depression.

Therapist: Perhaps before talking about the possible causes of your low mood, you can tell me more about what's going on.

Mr. III: The agitation has been replaced by depression. I'm crying in front of my kids. I'm nostalgic. I'm getting into bed at 8:30. I can't concentrate on a movie! I did get up for 2 days this week without the terror I've previously had, but I don't like what all this medicine is doing to me.

Therapist: Last week, you were grateful to have the lorazepam. I agree that you're depressed but you've been struggling with these symptoms for a long time, especially since your father's death.

Mr. III: This is beyond my father. Yeah, I've been thinking about him a lot and wearing his jewelry. I took my kid to my neighborhood where I grew up and showed her around. But this is beyond that. I was reading a book about these drugs. I know it can make you worse.

Therapist: What you've read is correct, though in my experience it's usually more of a theoretical concern than an actual one. You're taking a pretty low dose of lorazepam now [0.5 mg three times per day]. You can cut back, but we need to be careful that you do not have a reemergence of the marked agitation that you had a couple of weeks ago.

Mr. III: I think the Lexapro did that to me.

Therapist: The Lexapro is only part of the problem. I think it's really hard for you to depend upon me for help. You like being the one depended upon, not the other way around. I think it leaves you feeling out of control.

Mr. III: (annoyed) I never thought I would have to come here for so long. I know your intentions are good but I'm sick and tired of it all.

Mr. III prided himself on being self-sufficient and in control. His life's work involved taking care of disabled children, a group with whom he identified. His narcissistic vulnerability was heightened by his awareness that he needed the therapist's help. Further complicating matters was Mr. III's projection and displacement of his own anger onto the drugs: They were either weak and powerless or threatening to harm him. However, it was often impossible to determine how much of his complaint was a defensive distortion and how much was grounded in reality. This was difficult, in part, because the therapist's countertransference vulnerability was evoked with the repeated experience that Mr. III's criticisms were legitimate; that is, either the medication was not effective and/or intolerable side effects were being created.

These problems led to numerous medication changes, seeking to find the "magic bullet" without dealing explicitly with the patient's unrealistic expectations about medication and his devaluation of what was being offered. In this way, the therapist could be seen as participating in the patient's problems with compliance. As the therapist grasped Mr. III's fear of dependency, he was gradually able to help him observe the psychological root of his anxieties about the medication. It remained to be seen whether Mr. III could tolerate the dependency required to get better without resorting to paranoid defenses that would repeatedly undermine his and his therapist's best intentions.

THE PROBLEM OF SUBSTANCE ABUSE

Substance abuse complicates both pharmacologic and psychotherapeutic aspects of treatment. Major psychiatric illness—mood disorders, anxiety disorders, and psychotic conditions—as well as personality disorders have significant comorbidity with substance use/abuse (American Psychiatric Association, 1995). While an extensive discussion of this important topic is beyond the scope of this book, we will highlight common problems tied to substance abuse.

As noted in Hendin et al. (2006), clinicians engaged in an open-ended treatment may be at risk to assess and treat substance abuse inadequately. The psychodynamic therapist who does not actively inquire about drug use will risk missing the data necessary to identify the problem, since denial is a well-known defense for this patient population. The therapist may also wish to deny the presence of a significant abuse problem because to do otherwise requires an active, directive, and potentially limit-setting role—a posture with which many dynamic therapists are uncomfortable.

Therapists can also avoid dealing with the problem by rationalizing that they are addressing deeper issues that, once resolved, will ameliorate the substance-abuse problem. However, significant substance abuse not only interferes with a patient's ability to make use of psychotherapy but can also develop a life of its own and require an approach that treats it as a serious problem in its own right, while acknowledging important links to major psychiatric illness or personality disorders.

A recent review of controlled studies for alcohol-use disorders suggests that fostering insight may be of limited value compared to social-skills training, behavior contracting, brief interventions, or behavioral marital therapy (Miller & Wilbourne, 2002). Woody, McLellan, Luborsky, and O'Brien (1995) found the addition of dynamic therapy more effective than drug counseling alone for patients on methadone maintenance with significant psychiatric symptoms in addition to opiate abuse. Furthermore, many addictive states can respond, at least in part, to opiate antagonists and other agents (Amato et al., 2005; Buonopane & Petrakis, 2005). Patients should be informed about the available psychotherapeutic and pharmacologic options.

In evaluating the patient, the therapist should consider whether the substance use reflects an effort at self-medication. Khantzian (1985), who introduced the self-medication hypothesis of addictive disorders, suggested that drugs of abuse were not randomly chosen and were efforts to deal with painful affects. For example, a bipolar patient's addiction to cocaine can reflect an effort to minimize the lows and perpetuate the ego-syntonic state of hypomania. Opiates may be used in an effort to cope with overwhelming depression or anger. Alcohol is often employed in an effort to minimize anxiety, lift mood, and reduce insomnia. Substance abuse frequently exacerbates the very conditions the patient was hoping to manage, creating a vicious cycle.

Furthermore, the presence of significant substance use/abuse complicates the assessment of underlying psychiatric illness. Are the patient's symptoms due to substance use? Is the substance use an effort to treat symptoms? Is it a combination of both? If the patient can achieve abstinence, the therapist will be able to offer a clearer assessment of other conditions that may benefit from treatment. This two-step approach places an emphasis on abstinence as a prerequisite to clarifying diagnosis and treatment. Drugs that decrease craving as well as nondynamic therapies may be considered as adjuncts.

Some patients present with such clear symptoms of illness (often chronic depression) that the clinician will decide to cautiously begin a trial of an appropriate medication at the same time as encouraging abstinence. If ego functioning is not too impaired, the patient may be able to reflect on the underlying triggers for substance use. Sometimes, substance abuse becomes such a serious problem that more drastic steps, like hospitalization or residential treatment, must be considered. Occasionally, it is not until treatment is well under way that the therapist identifies a significant substance use/abuse problem.

Ms. GGG, discussed previously, initially acknowledged drinking only two glasses of wine per night and having no other substance-abuse problem. As she developed a psychotic depression, her substance abuse, which involved both alcohol and oxycodone, escalated. A combination of factors brought the problem to the attention of her analyst and pharmacotherapist. She accidentally injured herself after ingesting pain killers, incurring a visible wound on her head and requiring medical intervention. In addition, her escalating guilt during her depressive illness made it increasingly intolerable for her to withhold her substance-abuse problem from her therapists, and a positive therapeutic alliance had sufficiently taken hold for her to express her problem without fearing attack or rejection.

Once the problem was revealed, her psychoanalyst helped her to identify the triggers to her substance use. This typically involved an intolerance of painful affects tied to fears of abandonment and loss. Antidepressant and antipsychotic medication and intensive therapy helped her substantially, and she was able to achieve total abstinence from alcohol over a period of months. This was facilitated by attendance at Alcoholics Anonymous. She initially resisted AA but eventually found it to be a source of support when she found a sponsor with whom she could identify. She became largely abstinent from opiates, with only one slip when under extreme stress.

Technically, it was important that both her psychiatrist and analyst recommended an adjunctive treatment for her substance-abuse problem along with making that problem an explicit part of her psychotherapy. However, some patients may benefit from the ongoing involvement of a substance-abuse psychiatrist who can comfortably assume a more directive, prohibitive stance toward the patient's substance use, while the dynamic therapist continues to work in a more exploratory mode.

CAN MEDICATION UNDERMINE "INTEGRATION"?

Throughout this book we have emphasized the importance of a thoughtful and comprehensive approach to combined treatment with a focus on those conditions most frequently seen and treated by the psychodynamic clinician. The early biases against medication were based on the central role of affect and, more broadly, psychic pain as a motive force for an insight-oriented treatment. Are some patients better off without medication because its effectiveness forecloses psychotherapeutic exploration of issues deemed important for full recovery?

Swoiskin (2001) and Cabaniss (2001) have engaged in such a debate. Swoiskin asserts that there may be certain patients with primitive defenses (splitting, for example), who are prone to using medication to ward off owning parts of themselves. The very presence of medication makes it available to use as a fetishistic object, and the therapeutic effects can heighten the patient's conviction that his problems are caused by organic factors. Cabaniss counters that a patient's defensive structure is not a relevant consideration for determining the indication for medication, emphasizing the importance of a scientific, evidence-based approach. Furthermore, she encourages an ongoing curiosity about the meaning of the medication to the patient as a way of furthering an analytic process. In other words, resistance becomes grist for the mill. We concur with Cabaniss in this regard, while acknowledging that there are some patients who will decide that medication has been sufficiently helpful to curtail an introspective process that the therapist believes could have offered further benefit of integration.

Sometimes there are subtle effects of medication that seem to alter a patient's sense of integration in disturbing ways. Anecdotal reports of emotional blunting with SSRIs resonate with the experience of many clinicians who observe this state in patients who are otherwise euthymic. Hoehn-Saric et al. (1991) reported a case of frontal lobe syndrome (apathy, amotivation, emotional flatness) with fluoxetine. Opbroek et al. (2002), in a small open study of patients who had SSRI-induced sexual dysfunction, found that this population reported significantly less crying, irritation, care about other's feelings, sadness, erotic dreaming, creativity, surprise, anger, worry, sexual pleasure, and sexual interest. It is unknown how significant this problem is among all patients on SSRIs. However, there may be some situations where blunting can create the loss of a signal function with problematic consequences.

Ms. JJJ was an artist in her mid-20s who had been in combined treatment (weekly psychotherapy and venlafaxine) for major depression and longstanding masochistic character problems. In the fifth year of treatment, the therapist became concerned about a marked increase in irritability in response to minor injustices (a bus not stopping for her) and major ones (her boyfriend being inconsiderate). She was raised by a mother who frequently went into rages and by a father who encouraged the patient to "wear a smile" to calm the mother down or even apologize for misdeeds she had not done. At this point in the treatment, she lamented, "My lid is off. I feel like I have Tourette's." Her major complaints involved her boyfriend, whom she considered self-centered and inconsiderate.

After stopping venlafaxine and aborting a trial of a mood stabilizer (lamotrigine) due to side effects, the therapist decided to seek a second opinion. The consultant, while impressed by her irritability, felt that Ms. JJJ had spent much of her life accommodating to the needs of others and was angry because others did not readily accommodate to her. He felt this expectation needed to be examined as the next phase of therapy. The therapist, with the patient's consent, returned to fluoxetine (a drug she had found helpful but that may have caused weight gain) and her anger and irritability were markedly reduced. The relationship calmed down and her boyfriend proposed marriage. While the patient seemed excited about marriage, there continued to be hints of dissatisfaction. However, the fluoxetine made her less irritable and more attractive to her boyfriend.

The loss of irritability, however, also seemed to cause the loss of a signal function indicating her dissatisfaction had a basis in external reality. She married, soon became pregnant, and had a child. She presented 3 months postpartum worrying that she had a postpartum depression—a concern that was put to rest with careful examination. Upon exploration, she described her husband being verbally abusive toward her, complaining about how heavy she was postpartum. She also spoke of his drinking alcohol to excess—a problem that she observed existed long before she had married but had "buried."

While it appeared that the stress of parenthood had resulted in an escalation of her husband's behavior, the patient and therapist observed that a maternal transference was being enacted between the patient and the husband with the husband's behavior reminiscent of her mother's aggressive attacks against her. Additionally, the patient realized that the husband's behavior was not significantly different from that prior to marriage. It would be inappropriate to conclude that fluoxetine caused this state of affairs. However, the case suggests that the patient's masochistic tendencies (expressed by the decision to marry) may have been accentuated by the use of fluoxetine because the latter served to blunt the irritation and anger she had felt toward him.

CONCLUDING COMMENTS

Given the large number of patients suffering with major psychiatric illness, personality pathology, and substance abuse who seek treatment, it is not surprising that many of the patients we treat fall into the category of the complex case. A systematic assessment of how the clinician approaches his patient in delivering combined treatment can help to improve the likelihood of a positive outcome. Among the questions that the therapist can ask are:

- If a patient is actively suicidal, is he receiving adequate medication? If not, is his reluctance to accept medication being addressed? Is the patient or his family dictating the terms of the treatment? Is substance abuse present?
- If the treatment is stalled, does the lack of progress stem from an untreated or undertreated drug-repsonsive syndrome (an obstruction), dynamic issues (a resistance), or both? How is countertransference frustration affecting the therapist's assessment?
- If dynamic factors are involved in a stalled treatment, is this resistance related to a state of illness, trait personality, or some combination? Does this resistance have an impact on the patient's ability to receive adequate medication treatment?
- Is there an interaction between aspects of the patient's lack of progress that are best viewed as dynamic and those that are biological? If this is so, what is the primary intervention that needs to take place to end the stalemate? What are the ongoing simultaneous interventions that need to take place?
- Are there personality variables that have been inadequately identified that complicate the treatment course? Are these variables seen as existing on a dimension with the pharmacologically treated state or are they functioning as an independent variable?
- Is there a problem with substance use/abuse that has not been adequately addressed and is interfering with the psychotherapy or pharmacotherapy?
- Does the patient require an approach that has not yet been considered? Is the therapist too wedded to his way of working to consider other kinds of psychotherapy that are not primarily psychodynamic? Would the patient benefit from couples treatment, group psychotherapy, dialectical behavior therapy, or cognitive behavior therapy?

While being alert to the right questions to ask will not guarantee a successful treatment outcome, our hope is that by considering these questions the clinician will more likely optimize his care of the frequently encountered complex case.

References

Abel-Horowitz, J. (1998). Psychopharmacotherapy during an analysis. *Psychoanalytic Inquiry, 18,* 673–701.

Adelman, S. A. (1985). Pills as transitional objects: A dynamic understanding of the use of medication in psychotherapy. *Psychiatry, 48,* 246–253.

Akiskal, H. S. (2005). Preface. In M. Rosenbluth, S. Kennedy, & R. Bagby (Eds.), *Depression and personality: Conceptual and clinical challenges* (pp. xii–xvi). Washington, DC: American Psychiatric Publishing.

Akiskal, H. S., Hirshfeld, R. M., & Yerevanian, B. I. (1983). The relationship of personality to affective disorders. *Archives of General Psychiatry, 40,* 801–810.

Akiskal, H. S., Chen, S. E., Davis, G. E., Puzantian, V. R., Kashgarian, M., & Bolinger, J. M. (1985). Borderline: An adjective in search of a noun. *Journal of Clinical Psychiatry, 46,* 41–48.

Amato, L., Davoli, M., Perucci, C., Ferri, M., Gaggiano, F., & Mattick, R. (2005). An overview of systematic reviews of the effectiveness of opiate maintenance therapies: Available evidence to inform clinical practice and research. *Journal of Substance Abuse and Treatment, 28,* 321–329.

American Psychiatric Association. (1994). *Diagnostic and statistical manual of mental disorders* (4th ed.). Washington, DC: American Psychiatric Association.

American Psychiatric Association. (1995). Practice guidelines for the treatment of patients with substance use disorders: Alcohol, cocaine, opioids. *American Journal of Psychiatry* [suppl.], *152,* 1–80.

American Psychiatric Association. (1998). Practice guideline for the treatment of patients with panic disorder. *American Journal of Psychiatry* [suppl.], *155,* 1 34.

American Psychiatric Association. (2000). Practice guideline for the treatment of patients with major depressive disorder (revision). *American Journal of Psychiatry* [suppl.], *157,* 1–45.

American Psychiatric Association. (2001). Practice guideline for the treatment of patients with borderline personality disorder. *American Journal of Psychiatry* [10 suppl.], *158,* 1–52.

Awad, G. A. (2001). The effects of medication on the psychoanalytic process: The case of selective serotonin reuptake inhibitors. In *The psychoanalytic study of the child,* Vol. 56 (pp. 263–285). New Haven, CT: Yale University Press.

Barlow, D. H., Gorman, J. M., Shear, M. K., & Woods, S. W. (2000). Cognitive–behavioral therapy, imipramine, or their combination for panic disorder. *Journal of the American Medical Association, 283,* 2529–2536.

Barsky, A. J., Saintfort, R., Rogers, M. P., & Borus, J. F. (2002). Medication side effects and the nocebo phenomenon. *Journal of the American Medical Association, 287,* 622–627.

Baxter, L., Schwartz, M., Bergman, K. S., Szuba, M. P., Buze, B. M., Massiota, J.C., Mazraki, A., Sclin, C. E., Ferny, M., Munford, P., & Phelps, M. E. (1992). Caudate metabolic rate changes with both drug and behavior therapy for obsessive–compulsive disorder. *Archives of General Psychiatry, 49*, 681–689.

Bergman, M. S. (Ed.). (2000). *The Hartmann era*. New York: Other Press.

Bieling, P., & MacQueen, G. (2005). Bipolar disorder and personality: Constructs, findings, and challenges. In M. Rosenbluth, S. Kennedy, & R. Bagby (Eds.), *Depression and personality: Conceptual and clinical challenges* (pp. 187–228). Washington, DC: American Psychiatric Publishing.

Blatt, S. J. (2004). *Experiences of depression: Theoretical, clinical, and research perspectives*. Washington, DC: American Psychological Association.

Book, H. E. (1987). Some psychodynamics of noncompliance. *Canadian Journal of Psychiatry, 32*(2), 115–117.

Brandchaft, B. (2001). Obsessional disorders: A developmental systems perspective. *Psychoanalytic Inquiry, 21*(2), 253–288.

Buonopane, A., & Petrakis, I. L. (2005). Pharmacotherapy of alcohol use disorders. *Substance Use and Misuse, 40*, 1895–1897.

Busch, F. N. (1998). Prologue to "psychoanalysis and medication." *Psychoanalytic Inquiry, 18*, 603–605.

Busch, F. N., Cooper, A. M., Klerman, G. L., Shapiro, T. and Shear, M. K. (1991). Neurophysiological, cognitive-behavioral and psychoanalytic approaches to panic disorder: Toward an integration. *Psychoanalytic Inquiry* 11, 316–332.

Busch, F. N., & Gould, E. (1993). Transference/countertransference in the pharmacotherapy/psychotherapy triangle. *Hospital and Community Psychiatry, 44*, 772–774.

Busch, F. N., & Auchincloss, E. L. (1995). The psychology of prescribing and taking medication. In H. Schwartz, E. Bleiberg, & S. Weissman (Eds.), *Psychodynamic concepts in general psychiatry* (pp. 401–416). Arlington, VA: American Psychiatric Press.

Busch, F. N., Rudden, M. G., & Shapiro, T. (2004). *Psychodynamic treatment of depression*. Washington, DC: American Psychiatric Press.

Cabaniss, D. L. (1998). Shifting gears: The challenge to teach students to think psychodynamically and psychopharmacologically at the same time. *Psychoanalytic Inquiry, 18*, 639–656.

Cabaniss, D. L. (2001). Beyond dualism: Psychoanalysis and medication in the 21st century. *Bulletin of the Menninger Clinic, 65*, 160–170.

Cabaniss, D. L., & Roose, S. P. (2005). Psychoanalysis and psychopharmacology: New research, new paradigms. *Clinical Neuroscience Research, 4*, 399–403.

Caligor, E., Hamilton, M., Schneier, H., Donovan, J., & Roose, S. (2003). Converted versus clinic patients in the psychoanalytic training clinic: Implications for training. *Journal of the American Psychoanalytic Association, 51*, 201–220.

Cooper, A. M. (1985). Will neurobiology influence psychoanalysis? *American Journal of Psychiatry, 142*, 1395–1402.

Cornell, D. G. (1985). Psychoanalytic and biological perspectives on depression: Contradictory or complementary? *Psychoanalytic Psychology, 2*, 21–34.

Damasio, A. R. (1994). *Descartes' error*. New York: G. P. Putnam's Sons.

Deny, K. (1999). Evidence-based medicine and medical authority. *Journal of Medical Humanities, 20*, 247–263.

Docherty, J., Marder, S. R., Van Kammen, D. P., & Siris, S. G. (1977). Psychotherapy and pharmacotherapy: Conceptual issues. *American Journal of Psychiatry, 134*, 529–533.

Doidge, N., Simon, B., Brauer, L., Grant, D., First, M., Brunshaw, J., Lancee, W. J., Stevens, A., Oldham, J. M., & Mosher, P. (2002). Psychoanalytic patients in the U.S., Canada, and Australia: I. DSM-IIIR disorders, indications, previous treatment, medications, and length of treatment. *Journal of the American Psychoanalytical Association, 50*, 575–614.

Donovan, S. J., & Roose, S. P. (1995). Medication use during psychoanalysis: A survey. *Journal of Clinical Psychiatry, 56*, 177–178.

Dumit, J. (2003). Is it me or my brain? Depression and neuroscientific facts. *Journal of Medical Humanities, 24*, 35–47.

Eissler, K. (1953). The effect of the structure of the ego on psychoanalytic technique. *Journal of the American Psychoanalytic Association, 1*, 104–143.

Elliot, C., & Chambers, T. (Eds.) (2004). *Prozac as a way of life*. Chapel Hill: The University of North Carolina Press.

Esman, A. H. (1989). Psychoanalysis and general psychiatry: Obsessive–compulsive disorder as paradigm. *Journal of the American Psychoanalytical Association, 37*, 319–336.

Esman, A. H. (2001). Obsessive–compulsive disorder: Current views. *Psychoanalytic Inquiry, 21*(2), 145–156.

Fava, M., & Davidson, K. G. (1996). Definition and epidemiology of treatment-resistant depression. *Psychiatric Clinics of North America, 19*(2), 179–200.

Forrest, D. V. (2004), Elements of dynamics: II. Psychodynamic prescribing. *Journal of the American Academy of Psychoanalysis and Dynamic Psychiatry, 32*(2), 359–380.

Freud, S. (1909a). *Analysis of a phobia in a five-year-old boy*, standard edition, Vol. 10 (pp. 5–149). London: Hogarth Press, 1955.

Freud, S. (1909b). *Notes upon a case of obsessional neurosis*, standard edition, Vol. 1 (pp. 155–318). London: Hogarth Press, 1961.

Freud, S. (1916). *Some character types met with in psychoanalytic work*, standard edition, Vol. 14 (pp. 310–333). London: Hogarth Press, 1964.

Freud, S. (1940 [1938]). *An outline for psychoanalysis*, standard edition, Vol. 23 (pp. 144–207). London: Hogarth Press, 1964.

Friedman, R. C. (1991). The depressed masochistic patient: Diagnostic and management considerations—A contemporary psychoanalytic perspective. *Journal of the American Academy of Psychoanalysis, 19*, 9–30.

Friedman, R. C., Garrison, W. B., Bucci, W., & Gorman, B. S. (2005). Factors affecting change in private psychotherapy patients of senior psychoanalysts: An effectiveness study. *Journal of the American Academy of Psychoanalysis Dynamic Psychiatry, 33*, 583–610.

Gabbard, G. O. (1992). Psychodynamic psychiatry in the decade of the brain. *American Journal of Psychiatry, 149*, 991–998.

Gabbard, G. O. (1997). A reconsideration of objectivity in the analyst. *International Journal of Psychoanalysis, 78*, 15–26.

Gabbard, G. O. (2000). *Psychodynamic psychiatry in clinical practice* (3rd ed.). Washington, DC: American Psychiatric Press.

Gabbard, G. O. (2001). Psychoanalytically informed approaches to the treatment of obsessive–compulsive disorder. *Psychoanalytic Inquiry, 21*, 208–221.

Gabbard, G. O. (2005). Mind, brain, and personality disorders. *American Journal of Psychiatry, 162,* 648–655.

Gabbard, G. O., & Freedman, R. (2006). Psychotherapy in the journal: What's missing? *American Journal of Psychiatry, 163*(2), 182–184.

Gabbard, G. O., & Kay, J. (2001). The fate of integrated treatment: Whatever happened to the biopsychosocial psychiatrist? *American Journal of Psychiatry, 158,* 1956–1963.

Glick, R. A., & Roose, S. P. (2006). Talking about medication. *Journal of the American Psychoanalytic Association, 54,* 745–762.

Goldapple, K., Segal, Z., Carson, C., Lau, M., Bieling, P., Kennedy, S., & Mayberg, H. (2004). Modulation of cortical-limbic pathways in major depression. *American Journal of Psychiatry, 61,* 34–41.

Gorman, J. M., Kent, J. M., Sullivan, G. M., & Coplan, J. D. (2000). Neuroanatomical hypothesis of panic disorder, revised. *American Journal of Psychiatry, 157,* 493–505.

Gould, E., & Busch, F. N. (1998). Special issues in the psychopharmacology/psychotherapy triangle. *Psychoanalytic Inquiry, 18,* 730–745.

Greenacre, P. (1977). *Emotional growth,* Vol. 1. New York: International University Press.

Greene, M. (2001). Effects of medication on the psychoanalytic process: A case study. *Journal of the American Psychoanalytic Association, 49,* 607–628.

Gunderson, J. G., Weinberg, I., Daversa, M. T., Jueppenbender, K. D., Zanarini, M. C., Shea, M. T., Skodol, A. E., Sanislow, C. A., Yen, S., Morey, L. C., Grilo, C. M., McGlashan, T. H., Stout, R. L., & Dyck, I. (2006). Descriptive and longitudinal observations on the relationship of borderline personality disorder and bipolar disorder. *American Journal of Psychiatry, 163,* 1173–1178.

Guscott, R., & Grof, P. (1991). The clinical meaning of refractory depression: A review for the clinician. *American Journal of Psychiatry, 148,* 695–704.

Gutheil, T. G. (1982). The psychology of psychopharmacology. *Bulletin of the Menninger Clinic, 46,* 321–330.

Gwynn, N., & Roose, S. (2004). Medication management during psychoanalysis. *Journal of the American Psychoanalytic Association, 52,* 1243–1244.

Hartmann, H. (1939). *Ego psychology and the problem of adaptation* (D. Rappaport, Trans.). New York: International University Press, 1958.

Hausner, R. (1985). Medication and transitional phenomena. *International Journal of Psychoanalytic Psychotherapy, 11,* 375–398.

Hendin, H., Haas, A. P., Maltsberger, J. T., Koestner, B., & Szanto, K. (2006). Problems in psychotherapy with suicidal patients. *American Journal of Psychiatry, 163,* 67–72.

Hirschfeld, R. M. A. & Holzer. C. E. (1994). Depressive personality disorder: Clinical implications. *Journal of Clinical Psychiatry,* 55 (4, suppl.), 10–17.

Hoehn-Saric, R., Harris, G., Pearlson, G., Cox, C. S., Machlin, S. R., & Camargo, E. E. (1991). A fluoxetine-induced frontal lobe syndrome in an obsessive compulsive patient. *Journal of Clinical Psychiatry, 61,* 356–359.

Howland, R. H., & Thase, M. E. (2005). Refractory and chronic depression: The role of axis II disorders in assessment and treatment. In M. Rosenbluth, S. H. Kennedy, & R. M. Bagby (Eds.), *Depression and personality: Conceptual and clinical challenges* (pp. 157–186). Washington, DC: American Psychiatric Publishing.

Jackson, S. (1992). The listening healer in the history of psychological healing. *American Journal of Psychiatry, 149,* 1623–1632.

Jacobs, T. J. (2001). On unconscious communication and covert enactments: Some reflections on their role in the analytic situation. *Psychoanalytic Inquiry, 21,* 4–23.

Janicek, P. G., Davis, J. M., Preskorn, S. H. and Ayd, F. A. (2006). *Principles and practice of psychopharmacotherapy.* Philadelphia: Lippincott Williams & Wilkins.

Kahn, D. A. (1991). Medication consultation and split treatment during psychotherapy. *Journal of the American Academy of Psychoanalysis, 19,* 84–98.

Kandel, E. R. (1979). Psychotherapy and the single synapse. *New England Journal of Medicine, 308,* 1028–1037.

Kandel, E. R. (1999). Biology and the future of psychoanalysis: A new intellectual framework for psychiatry revisited. *American Journal of Psychiatry, 156,* 505–524.

Kantor, S. (1990). Depression: When is psychotherapy not enough? *Psychiatric Clinics of North America, 13,* 241–254.

Keller, M. B., McCullough, J. P., Klein, D. N., Arnow, B., Dunner, D. L., Gelenberg, A. J., Markowitz, J. C., Nemeroff, C. B., Russell, J. M., Thase, M. E., Trivedi, M. H., & Zajecka, J. (2000). A comparison of nefazodone, the cognitive–behavioral system of psychotherapy, and their combination for the treatment of chronic depression. *New England Journal of Medicine, 342,* 1462–1470.

Kelly, K. V. (1998). Principles, pragmatics, and parameters in clinical analysis: The dilemma of pharmacotherapy. *Psychoanalytic Inquiry, 18,* 716–729.

Kendler, K. S. (2005). Toward a philosophical structure for psychiatry. *American Journal of Psychiatry, 162,* 433–440.

Khantzian, E. J. (1985). The self-medication hypothesis of addictive disorders: Focus on heroin and cocaine dependence. *American Journal of Psychiatry, 142,* 1259–1264.

Klerman, G. L. (1988). Depression and related disorders of mood (affective disorders). In A. M. Nicholi (Ed.), *The new Harvard guide to psychiatry* (pp. 309–336). Cambridge: Harvard University Press.

Klerman, G. L. (1990). The psychiatric patient's right to effective treatment: Implications of *Osheroff v. Chestnut Lodge. American Journal of Psychiatry, 147,* 409–418.

Kocsis, J. H., Frances, A. J., Voss, C., Mann, J. J., Mason, B. J., & Sweeney, J. (1988). Imipramine treatment of chronic depression. *Archives of General Psychiatry, 45,* 253–257.

Kocsis, J. H., Friedman, R. A., Markowitz, J. C., Leon, A. C., Miller, N. L., Gniwesch, L., & Parides, M. (1996). Maintenance therapy for chronic depression: A controlled clinical trial of desipramine. *Archives of General Psychiatry, 53,* 769–774.

Kramer, P. (1993). *Listening to Prozac.* New York: Penguin Books.

LaFarge, L. (2000). Interpretation and containment. *International Journal of Psychoanalysis, 81,* 67–84.

Leahy, R. L., McGinn, L. K., Busch, F. N., & Milrod, B. L. (2005). Anxiety disorders. In G. O. Gabbard, J. S. Beck, & J. Holmes (Eds.), *Oxford textbook of psychotherapy* (pp. 137–162). Oxford: Oxford University Press.

LeDoux, J. E. (1996). *The emotional brain: The mysterious underpinnings of emotional life.* New York: Simon and Schuster.

Levenson, E. A. (2006). Response to John Steiner. *International Journal of Psychoanalysis, 87,* 321–324.

Lipton, M. A. (1983). Editorial: A letter from Anna Freud. *American Journal of Psychiatry, 140,* 1583–1584.

Malin, B. (1998). Epilogue to the issue: Psychoanalysis and medication. *Psychoanalytic Inquiry, 18,* 746–762.

Maltsberger, J. T., & Buie, D. H. (1974). Countertransference hate in the treatment of suicidal patients. *Archives of General Psychiatry, 30,* 625–633.

Mayberg, H., Liotti, M., Brannan, S. K., McGinnis, S., Mahurin, R. K., Jerabek, P. A., Silva, J. A., Tekell, J. L., Martin, C. C., Lancaster, J. L., & Fox, P. T. (1999). Reciprocal limbic-cortical function and negative mood: Converging PET findings in depression and normal sadness. *American Journal of Psychiatry, 156,* 675–682.

Mayberg, H., Silva, J. A., Brannan, S. K., Tekell, J. L., Mahurin, R. K., McGinnis, S., & Jerabek, P. A. (2002). The functional neuroanatomy of the placebo effect. *American Journal of Psychiatry, 159,* 728–737.

McDermut, W., Zimmerman, M., & Chelminski, I. (2003). The construct validity of depressive personality disorder. *Journal of Abnormal Psychology, 112,* 49–60.

Meares, R. (2001). A specific developmental deficit in obsessive–compulsive disorder: The example of the wolf man. *Psychoanalytic Inquiry, 21*(2), 289–319.

Metzl, J. M., & Riba, M. (2003). Understanding the symbolic value of medications: A brief review. *Primary Psychiatry, 10,* 45–48.

Miller, W. R., & Wilbourne, P. L. (2002). Mesa Grande: A methodological analysis of clinical trials of treatments for alcohol use disorders. *Addiction, 97,* 265–277.

Milrod, B. L., & Busch, F. N. (1998). Combining psychodynamic psychotherapy with medication in the treatment of panic disorder: Exploring the dynamic meaning of medication. *Psychoanalytic Inquiry, 18,* 702–715.

Milrod, B. L., Busch, F. N., Cooper, A. M., & Shapiro T. (1997). *Manual of panic-focused psychodynamic psychotherapy.* Washington, DC: American Psychiatric Press, 1997.

Milrod, B. L., Leon, A. C., Busch, F. N., Rudden, M., Schwalberg, M., Clarkin, J., Aronson, A., Singer, M., Turchin, W., Klass, E. T., Graf, E., Teres, J. J., & Shear, M. K. (2007). A randomized controlled clinical trial of psychoanalytic psychotherapy for panic disorder. *American Journal of Psychiatry,* 164 (2), 265–272.

Mintz, D. (2002). Meaning and medication in the care of treatment-resistant patients. *American Journal of Psychotherapy, 56,* 322–338.

Noblett, K. L., & Coccaro, E. F. (2005). The psychobiology of personality disorders. In M. Rosenbluth, S. Kennedy, & R. Bagby (Eds.), *Depression and personality: Conceptual and clinical challenges* (pp. 19–42). Washington, DC: American Psychiatric Publishing.

Oldham, J. M. (2006). Integrated treatment for borderline personality disorder. *Psychiatric Annals, 36*(5), 361–369.

Opbroek, A., Delgado, P. L., Laukes, C., McGahuey, C., Katsanis, J., Moreno, F. A., & Manber, R. (2002). Emotional blunting associated with SSRI-induced sexual dysfunction. Do SSRIs inhibit emotional responses? *International Journal of Neuropsychopharmacology, 5,* 147–151.

Ostow, M. (1962). *Drugs in psychoanalysis and psychotherapy.* New York: Basic Books.

PDM Taskforce. (2006). *Psychodynamic diagnostic manual*. Silver Spring, MD: Alliance of Psychoanalytic Organizations.

Pollock, G. H. (1986). Do multiple psychological diseases exist simultaneously? *Annual Review of Psychoanalysis, 14*, 143–146.

Preston, G. A., Marchant, B. K., Reimherr, F. W., Strong, R. E., & Hedges, D. W. (2004). Borderline personality disorder in patients with bipolar disorder and response to lamotrigine. *Journal of Affective Disorders, 79*, 297–303.

Riba, M.B., & Tasman, A. (2006). Psychodynamic perspectives in combining therapies. *Psychiatric Annals, 36*(5), 353–360.

Roose, S. P. (1990). The use of medication in combination with psychoanalytic psychotherapy or psychoanalysis. In R. Michels (Ed.), *Psychiatry* (pp. 1–9). Philadelphia: J. B. Lipincott.

Roose, S. P. (1995). Does anxiety obstruct or motivate treatment? When to talk, when to prescribe and when to do both. In S. P. Roose & R. E. Glick (Eds.), *Anxiety as symptom and signal* (pp. 155–169). Hillsdale, NJ: The Analytic Press.

Roose, S. P., & Gabbard, G. O. (1997). Resistance to medication during psychoanalysis. *Journal of Psychotherapy Practice and Research, 6*, 239–248.

Roose, S. P., & Johannet, C. (1998). Medication and psychoanalysis: Treatments in conflict. *Psychoanalytic Inquiry, 18*, 606–620.

Roose, S. P., & Stern, R. H. (1995). Medication use in training cases: A survey. *Journal of the American Psychoanalytic Association, 43*, 163–170.

Ryder, A. G., Bagby, R. M., & Schuller, D. R. (2002). The overlap of depressive personality disorder and dysthymia: A categorical problem with a dimensional solution. *Harvard Review of Psychiatry, 10*, 337–352.

Sackheim, H. A. (2001). The definition and meaning of treatment-resistant depression. *Journal of Clinical Psychiatry* [suppl. 16], *62*, 10–17.

Sandberg, L. S. (1998). Analytic listening and the act of prescribing medication. *Psychoanalytic Inquiry, 18*, 621–638.

Sarwer-Foner, G. J. (1983). An overview of combined psychopharmacology and psychotherapy. In M. H. Greenhill & A. Gralnick (Eds.), *Psychopharmacology and psychotherapy* (pp. 165–180). New York: Macmillan.

Schlierf, C. (1983). Transitional objects and object relationship in a case of anxiety neurosis. *International Review of Psychoanalysis, 110*, 319–332.

Shear, M. K., Cooper, A. M., Klerman, G. L., Busch, F. N. and Shapiro, T. (1993). A psychodynamic model of panic disorder. *American Journal of Psychiatry*, 150, 859–866.

Siever, L., & Davis, K. (1991). A psychobiological perspective on the personality disorders. *American Journal of Psychiatry, 148*, 1647–1658.

Silverman, D. K. (2005). What works in psychotherapy and how do we know? What evidence-based practice has to offer. *Psychoanalytic Psychology, 22*, 306–312.

Steiner, J. (2006). Interpretive enactments and the analytic setting. *International Journal of Psychoanalysis, 87*, 315–320.

Stone, A. A. (1990). Law, science, and psychiatric malpractice: A response to Klerman's indictment of psychoanalytic psychiatry. *American Journal of Psychiatry, 147*, 419–427.

Suomi, S. J. (2003). Gene–environment interactions and the neurobiology of social conflict. *Annals of the New York Academy of Science*, 1008, 132–139.

Swoiskin, M. (2001). Psychoanalysis and medication: Is real integration possible? *Bulletin of the Menninger Clinic, 65,* 143–159.

Thase, M. E. (2000). Psychopharmacology in conjunction with psychotherapy. In R. Ingram & R. C. Snyder (Eds.), *Handbook of psychological change: Psychotherapy process and practices for the 21st century* (pp. 474–497). New York: Wiley.

Thase, M. E. (2003). Conceptual and empirical basis for integrating psychotherapy and pharmacotherapy. In B. Beitman, B. Blinder, M. Thase, M. Riba, & D. Safer (Eds.), *Integrating psychotherapy and pharmacotherapy* (pp. 111–140). New York: W. W. Norton.

Thase, M. E., & Howland, R. (1994). Refractory depression: Relevance of psychosocial factors and therapies. *Psychiatric Annals, 24,* 232–240.

Thase, M. E., Greenhouse, J. B., Frank, E., Reynolds, C. F., III, Pilkonis, P. A., Hurley, K., Grochinski, V., & Kupfer, D. J. (1997). Treatment of major depression with psychotherapy or psychotherapy–pharmacotherapy combinations. *Archives of General Psychiatry, 54,* 1009–1015.

Tillman, J. G. (2006). When a patient commits suicide: An empirical study of psychoanalytic clinicians. *International Journal of Psychoanalysis, 87,* 159–177.

Tutter, A. (2006). Medication as object. *Journal of the American Psychoanalytic Association, 54,* 781–804.

Wender, P. (1995). *Attention-deficit hyperactivity disorder in adults.* New York: Oxford University Press.

Winnocott, D. W. (1953). Transitional objects and transitional phenomena. *International Journal of Psychoanalysis, 34,* 89–97.

Woody, G. E., McLellan, A. T., Luborsky, L., & O'Brien, C. P. (1995). Psychotherapy in community methadone programs: A validation study. *American Journal of Psychiatry, 152,* 1302–1308.

Wright, J.H., & Hollifield, M. (2006). Guest editorial: Combining pharmacotherapy & psychotherapy. *Psychiatric Annals, 36*(5), 302–305.

Wurtzel, E. (1995). *Prozac nation: Young and depressed in America.* New York: Riverhead Press.

Wylie, H. W., & Wylie, M. L. (1995). Resistances and obstructions: Their distinction in psychoanalytic treatment. *Journal of Clinical Psychoanalysis, 4,* 185–207.

Wylie, H. W., & Wylie, M. L. (1996). "Bright spot": Technical recommendations concerning a phenomenon observed when combining psychoanalysis and medication. *Journal of Clinical Psychoanalysis, 5,* 553–559.

Yang, S., Caligor, E., Cabaniss, D. L., Luber, B., Donovan, J., Rosen, P., Forand, N. R., & Roose, S. P. (2004). Post-termination contact: A survey of prevalence, characteristics, and analyst attitudes. *Journal of the American Psychoanalytic Association, 52,* 455–457.

Zimmerman, M., Chelminski, I., & Posternak, M. A. (2005). Generalizability of antidepressant efficacy trials: Differences between depressed psychiatric outpatients who would or would not qualify for an efficacy trial. *American Journal of Psychiatry, 162,* 1370–1372.

Index

C